THE GOSPEL IMPERATIVE IN THE MIDST OF AIDS

Edited by Robert H. Iles

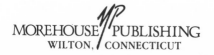

MOREHOUSE PUBLISHING
WILTON, CONNECTICUT

Morehouse Publishing
78 Danbury Road
Wilton, Connecticut 06897

Library of Congress Cataloging-in-Publication Data

The Gospel imperative in the midst of AIDS / edited by
  Robert H. Iles.
     p.   cm.
  Bibliography: p.
  ISBN 0-8192-1505-8
  1. AIDS (Disease)—Religious aspects—Christianity—Congresses.
I. Iles, Robert H., 1938–
RA644.A25G67   1990
261.8'321969792—dc20   89-12295
                                                              CIP

Printed in the United States of America
by
BSC LITHO
Harrisburg, PA

Dedication

This book is dedicated to Armando Rios, whose life on this planet was ended by death as a consequence of AIDS on July 9, 1989. In life he was a bridge between those infected with HIV and those not infected; between Hispanic and Anglo; between those of faith and those who despaired. Over that bridge love and compassion freely flowed. May he move from strength to strength in the life of perfect service to the God whom he loved and worshipped.

Contents

Acknowledgments

This book is a product of an invitational symposium held at Church Divinity School of the Pacific in November 1988. The expenses of that symposium were underwritten by many people, whose support I wish to acknowledge.

The following bishops of the Episcopal Church were sponsors: Edmond Lee Browning, Frederick H. Borsch, William E. Swing, David Johnson, C. O. Schofield, William G. Burrill, David B. Birney, R. M. Anderson, William A. Jones, and George Bates. Other sponsors were the Episcopal Dioceses of Oklahoma and Washington, and the Parish of St. Mary the Virgin, San Francisco. The Standing Committee of the Diocese of South West Florida sponsored the symposium in memory of their late Bishop, Paul Haynes. Other sponsors were the Reverends Joe M. Doss, Kathleen Dale Roffina, Daniel P. Matthews, Stuart P. Coxhead, the Very Reverends John C. Sanders and William S. Pregnall, and the Rev. Canon Earl L. Conner of the National Episcopal AIDS Coalition. We are also grateful for the sponsorship of Gary John Fowler and Stephen Miller, both of the Diocese of Los Angeles.

Funding was also obtained from the following donors, whose support I gratefully acknowledge: Charity Weymouth, Lois J. Wolf, Bette C. Bordin, Steven Giovangelo, Joel T. Keys, Harry Pritchett, John C. Powers, Stephen McWhorter, Charles Carter, George McClaren, Edward M. Sunderland, Arthur S. Lloyd, the Parish of St. John-in-Montclair, Oakland, California. The following bishops also contributed: Robert L. Ladehoff, Paul Moore, Donald Hulstrand, Duncan Gray, Richard Grein, Donald P. Hart, Edward MacBurney, William Sanders, Allen L. Bartlett, Shannon Mallory, O'Kelley Whitaker, Victor M. Rivera, Leigh A. Wallace, S. B. Hulsey, John M. Krum, G. R. Millard, and David Henry Lewis, Jr.

The following individuals have contributed their creative energy to the symposium, serving as members of the planning committees, advisors, and staff: Jerry Anderson, Hobart Banks, Thad Bennett, William Barcus, Marian Cedarblade, Lynne Coggi, Earl Conner, David Cunningham, William Doubleday, Edward Franks, Blair Hatt, Deborah Hines, April Hockett, Richard Holdridge, Bonnie Hunter-Elliott, T. G. Jones, Mwalimu Imara, Holly McAlpen, Weston Miliken, Kathy O'Reilly, Patricia Page, Dolly Patterson, Eric Scharf, Ed Sunderland, Oliver Vannorsdall, and Lorentho Wooden.

I wish to express my gratitude to Linda Gulker for reading the manuscript and making helpful comments. Ann Lammers also supplied me with wise and skillful editorial counsel. I am grateful to Meg George for providing the computer/word processor upon which the manuscript was prepared. Ed Sunderland fed sheets of paper, soggy from firefighter's hoses, through a photocopier, salvaging the only copy of the manuscript after the computer and floppy disks containing the text had been destroyed by fire. He carries my undying gratitude.

Finally, and perhaps most fulsomely, I express my gratitude to Albert J. Ogle, the executive director of the All Saints/AIDS Service Center, for his vision and matchless developmental talents. He joins me in expressing gratitude to George F. Regas, the rector of All Saints Parish, his staff of clergy and laypeople of grace and great competence, and the members of the congregation of All Saints/Pasadena, who have supported the development of a ministry in response to the AIDS crisis, without reservation, and with great generosity.

Robert H. Iles

Preface

AIDS has created a spiritual crisis, and the issues this spiritual crisis raises comprise the central theme of this book. In the AIDS experience, Christians are confronted with questions that reach to the foundations of our humanity, our relationship to God and to each other. What does it mean to be the Church? What is the meaning of human life? What is the meaning of death? When my life is severely foreshortened, how do I choose to spend my time? That AIDS is renewing the Church is the *leitmotif* that sounds in every chapter of this book.

Ninety people gathered at the Church Divinity School of the Pacific in Berkeley, California, in November 1988 for a weekend of sharing and reflection on the Church's response to the epidemic of Acquired Immune Deficiency Syndrome (AIDS), the disease that has afflicted the United States since the early months of the decade and other countries, notably Africa, since the early 1970s. Six of those attending had been invited to address key themes and nine others to reflect on the papers that were distributed prior to the symposium. All invited to speak were leaders in the Church's response to AIDS.

This book reproduces these contributions as well as parts of the ensuing discussion by other participants. Several articles were submitted to the editor immediately following the weekend, and portions of these also are included. The symposium was directed to Episcopalians, as the organizers intend the project to be utilized as an educational resource for our own church. Most attending were Episcopalians; however, people joined us from several other denominations including Roman Catholics, Presbyterians, and Lutherans. We are grateful for the participation of the other church representatives and will be happy if others find the book useful as well.

The Church and AIDS

Why did a symposium dedicated to the AIDS experience seem

necessary? Some church members have asked, "Why AIDS masses? Shouldn't we have influenza masses? Or cancer masses? Why not masses for the common cold?" Those who read this book will hear several answers to these questions. The AIDS epidemic is a crisis, but (to use the old cliché) it is also an opportunity, perhaps of greater magnitude than we have seen previously. AIDS is shaking, changing, and reforming our society, forcing us to review our values, to deepen our faith, to change operative assumptions about our lives and relationship to God. Society is being required to change its health care delivery systems and to revise the way we pay for health care. The AIDS experience affects not only the people who are sick and their extended families but, just as importantly, the values of the human race and its constituent cultures.

This book has then as its major goal the task of doing theology: As we are ill with AIDS, what can we learn about God? What does God want of the People of God in response to those who live with this disease? As we "seek and serve Christ in all persons," and "strive for justice and peace among all people, and respect the dignity of every human being," what do we learn about God and the divine purpose for us?[1]

The experience of human contact and the emotional and spiritual support the participants offered to each other that November weekend were powerful. Those who provide care to persons with AIDS (PWAs) do so at a high risk of burnout. To understand this situation, note, for example, the statement of Ted Karpf, founder of the Dallas-AIDS Interfaith Network, that he had conducted funeral services for sixty persons who have died as a result of AIDS. What does this mean for him? We can estimate that he provided pastoral care to two to five people associated with each of the deceased persons. Additionally, approximately one hundred persons ill with the disease, each with friends and family, turned to him for pastoral care.

Was Ted Karpf simply dealing with the usual grieving process that accompanies death and illness? Of course not. He was responding to and caring for people who were socially marginalized: Many were persons whose sexual life-styles are not acceptable in mainstream America. Many were estranged from their families, both families of origin and, in some situations, spouses and children. Those ill were in the prime of life, ranging from age twenty through age forty. Many were using illegal drugs; possibly emotional difficulties preceded their use of narcotics. Each had a disease for which no cure is known. Karpf dealt with discrimination in its most egregious forms. He had to find his way through a maze of medical protocols, social policies regarding health care, and civil codes (or their absence) regulating discrimination. The people who received his care needed services from physicians, dentists, nurses, nursing homes, and morticians who often were reluctant or unwilling to provide these to persons with AIDS and their families. Often PWAs became unemployed soon after diagnosis and for support were dependent upon private insurance in some lucky cases or, more likely, government programs. Many had to wait for months before benefits were available. During this time they usually had no income. Often they were too ill and debilitated to stand in line at the Social Security office to fill out the endless forms. Ted Karpf was providing his ministry in a nation whose president refused even to speak publicly about AIDS, or acknowledge that there was a problem, during the first five years of his administration. This complex of emotionally charged factors requires far more from caregivers than other circumstances of illness and death.

Why This Book?

However, *The Gospel Imperative in the Midst of AIDS* is not about the day-to-day care of and ministry to PWAs. There is an ample supply of resources describing how to provide care in the AIDS crisis: many are listed in the bibliography. Further, this is not a "recipe book" for educating congregations about the AIDS crisis. That function is served by the parish study guide, [title]. Rather, this book provides theological grounding for inquiring minds in the Church. It raises questions, sometimes provocative questions, and provides a thoughtful context for those who recognize the need to respond but may not have clarified their own thinking about the complex, controversial, frequently inflammatory issues that surround the AIDS experience. In this book, discerning people struggle with these questions; many readers may disagree with their answers. At the very least we have attempted to provide a forum for discussion that allows for divergent views.

Reading This Book

This book is about a world crisis and the Church's response to it. But crises happen to people and are best understood through their eyes. The first chapter is by a man who is a priest and a person with AIDS. William Barcus has served in multiple capacities: as an advocate to the Church on behalf of PWAs, as a hands-on caregiver, and as a person living a relatively long time with AIDS. He was one of the designers and planners of the weekend dialogue but was too ill to be present. He provides a perspective on the AIDS experience that few can give.

Mwalimu Imara, a priest, a thanatologist, an ethicist, a civil rights leader, and a spokesperson for black Americans, responds to Barcus' passionate plea. The AIDS issue is inextricably intertwined with issues of personhood and discrimination against people of color, in our nation and throughout the world.

The introductions to part 2 and each subsequent part refine and sample the discussion that took place in Berkeley. As the papers had been made available to the participants in advance, most of the discussion time was spent responding to them.

Though originally these responses were made *after* the papers were presented, readers of this book will find they work well as introductions to the material. To convey the sense of immediacy that energizes any discussion, everyones' comments have been left in the present tense. In these introductions you will also read the extemporaneous comments of persons representing minority communities, set apart to give them weight and distinction. They have been reported with minimal editing, to convey to the reader (to the extent possible in the written word) the flavor and nuances of the speaker. I believe these comments call for the most sensitive and attuned reading and responses.

Part 2 is more explicitly theological, although theology is implicit throughout all the pages of this book. The question that must be answered anew each day of our lives is explored: What does it mean to be the Church? That question and the answer given in each time, each place, each circumstance, must precede and inform concrete and strategic discussion of issues. As there are many voices in this book (and in the AIDS experience in general), there are many views. But when Christians deliberate corporately, as the Body of Christ, we must attempt to see the issues through the eyes of Christ and act from that particular perspective.

Human sexuality is the next theme explored. In the United States, and this is unique to our country, between 60 and 80 percent of PWAs, depending upon the region, are homosexual in orientation, a circumstance that bluntly and unavoidably demands that the Church wrestle with human sexuality. I always have found religion, sex, and politics, the three subjects no "polite dinner guest" would ever bring up, to be the most interesting. AIDS allows us no alternative! If we are to be the Body of Christ in this era of our nation's history, we must deal with religion, sexuality, and public policy. I view this as an exciting opportunity!

The fourth part of *The Gospel Imperative in the Midst of AIDS* is titled "Sin and Sickness/Faith and Health," and even this title is controversial. Phyllis Leppert, a physician and churchwoman, has problems with the connection of faith to health and sin to sickness. Christ sent his followers into the world to proclaim the gospel *and* to heal. The Church cannot avoid its healing mission as it responds to a lethal epidemic.

The next area examined is death and loss. American Christians are, I believe, bicultural. While most twentieth-century Americans spend tremendous energy avoiding the reality of death, the Christian understanding of death is different. The secular culture attempts to deny the reality of death; the Christian culture says, with Paul, I want to live to be able to serve Christ, and I want to die to be with Christ. The Christian culture must be always on the attack against the denial of death. The AIDS crisis requires us to reaffirm the Christian understanding of death and dying.

Finally, in "Transformation: Visions and Plans," our contributors look forward. The Christian religion is by its nature eschatalogical, facing "end times," and readers are invited to look beyond sex, sickness, and death to an optimistic outcome as the book draws to a close.

The Gospel Imperative in the Midst of AIDS is dialogical, intending to stimulate discussion and learning in the Church. Denial of reality is death-oriented: The reality of AIDS is deadly to physical health and the body, but the denial of this crisis is deadly to the soul, not only the souls of infected and affected persons, but also to our entire society. God was in Christ, reconciling the world. The Church is the Body of Christ, and our mission is healing, the healing of mind, body, and soul. God is with us.

Robert H. Iles

Reference

1. *The Book of Common Prayer* (New York: Church Hymnal Corporation, 1979), from the Baptismal Covenant, p. 305.

Biographical Note

Robert H. Iles is a priest of the Episcopal Diocese of Los Angeles. He has served several parishes in that diocese and since 1973 has conducted a private practice in psychotherapy. He was the first western regional chair of the American Association of Sex Educators, Counselors, and Therapists and has taught human sexuality at the college level since 1973. He earned his theological degree at the Episcopal Theological Seminary in Virginia and has studied at the University of California at Los Angeles, the California Graduate Institute, the Graduate School of the Claremont Colleges, and the Kinsey Institute for Sex Research. He is at present a member of the faculty of Art Center College of Design and on the staff of All Saints Church in Pasadena. He was the founder and now serves as a member of the board of the All Saints/AIDS Service Center.

Part 1.
The Gospel Alive

The Gospel Imperative
William Henry Barcus III

Occasionally in human history great clouds pass over us that, with all their lightning, thunder, and darkness, become litmus tests for the human race. Acquired Immune Deficiency Syndrome (AIDS) is precisely such a litmus test. To humanity the question posed is, "Will you stay humane?" For the Church, with its curious mixture of humanity's worst and best, the AIDS crisis is a challenge to raise ourselves toward the Divine, for that is what we call the more humane. Or will the Church cling with unquestioning and easy adherence to the beliefs and dictates of earlier, primordial times? AIDS is a litmus test for all—in San Francisco, St. Louis, New York, Westchester, Washington, Zaire, Stockholm, Nashville—a test for men, women, straight, gay, black, white, Latino, the Asian community. Perhaps a parable can shed light on the nature of the test.

A series of photographs in *Life* magazine's issue of March 14, 1944, prompted the biggest avalanche of letters that *Life* had ever received. The photos showed red foxes in Holmes County, Ohio, who lived in the woods and ate mostly mice and crickets but also chicken and quail. This, the story explained, "made the brave men of Holmes County angry, because they wanted to kill the quail themselves." One Saturday morning about six hundred men, women, and children formed a big circle five miles across. They carried sticks and started to walk through woods and fields, yelling and baying to frighten the foxes, young and old, out of their holes. Inside this shrinking circle the foxes ran to and fro, tired and frightened. Sometimes a fox would, in its anger, dare to snarl back and be killed on the spot for its temerity. Sometimes one would stop in anguish and try to lick the hand of a tormenter. It, too, would be killed.

Sometimes, the photos showed, other foxes would stop to stay with their own wounded and dying. Finally, as the circle narrowed down to a few yards across, the few remaining foxes went to the center and laid down, not knowing what else to do. The men and the women knew; they hit the defeated animals with their clubs until they were dead, or they showed their children how to do it. This is a true story that *Life* reported as it happened in Holmes County. The good Christian people of Holmes County considered it sport.

I write as one wounded myself, weary from running, and say to the churches—the churches first, then the government, and then the world—"What have you done to my people? What have you done to your own people, your beautiful people, so swift and beautiful and bright?"

I see in those who have died, in those dying around me, more courage, forgiveness, nobility, more of God than I ever do in those who hate and hound and judge, those who have made so many want now "only to lay down and die." My people are being destroyed—and your people and all our people—not only by an illness called AIDS, but by a darker illness called hatred, which permitted AIDS to spread rampantly across all groups while administrations sat silent.

Would our brothers and sisters in the black community see their experience in this parable? Our Jewish friends? I assure you it is the experience of your brothers and sisters, sons and daughters, who happen to be born gay or who happen to be poor, who happen to be socially and educationally deprived. It is the experience of those whose parents abandon them, those who know kindness only from caregivers on the hospital wards to which they are consigned.

The Original Mission Statement of the Church

The God to whom I address my anguish, Job-like, is the same God to whom we all ultimately go home, to whom we all will answer. This same God, hoping to be seen at last clearly and experienced as the bridge between the Divine and the human, said to Simon Peter, "Simon Peter, lovest thou me? Feed my sheep."

There, in that imperative, was the Church's founding commission. There has never been a more powerful, revising-of-other-agendas mission. Leaping across all the ancient assembled concepts of the gods who were judgmental, we arrive at the face-to-face viewing. Clearly now we know what God is really like: compassionate and understanding, validating and affirming, standing always with the outcast, worrying less about the frailties in every life-style and more about the legalism, the hypocrisies that cause hearts to break.

"Simon Peter, lovest thou me?"

"You know I do, Lord."

"Then feed my sheep."

In that imperative to be a shepherd to the flock is our founding moral rock, our Church's mission statement to be lived out until the end of time. Transforming old hatred, old codes, old covenants is the new covenant, the new understanding, the new imperative, the new possibility offered by God to humankind in all our societal needs.

With those words to Peter, the Church was called into her very being as shepherd. In this imperative and commission to love and support others, Christ gave us a summation and a decoding of what the old moralistic legalizations struggled to discover. He gave us a moral approach that transcends the mores and cultural attitudes of any age. He gave us, finally, a moral rule for all time that can rewrite history's calamities whenever rediscovered and utilized: *We are to love our neighbor!*

That a good shepherd would leave behind, or ignore, those of his sheep who are ill or dying is unthinkable. To those in the churches who suppose AIDS is a human dilemma they can sit out, I say, "Hear the gospel." The Church is not to permit her flock to be attacked or isolated. Nor is she to turn into a ravaging wolf herself. To those in this country on the religious far Right who have held this nation's administration captive in bigoted sway, I say, "Hear the gospel!" Better to take the stakes out of your own eyes than to look so nervously at the slivers in the eye of your neighbor.

I call the Church to return boldly to her shepherding, as people seek counsel on "where to turn." I call her to do that quickly. People are dying. We do not have time to play with lives nor to play with our own souls.

Our AIDS-Generated Blind Spots

We will never see beyond our stakes, slivers, and blind spots if we do not critically examine them. In a nutshell, they are four:

1. Wanting to play god and sit in judgment on each other.
2. Misunderstanding what sin really is.
3. Seeing homosexuality as a condition assumed to be equated with sin.

4. Denying our children's vulnerability.

In our mad rush to judge, we ignore Jesus' commandment that we never again are to presume to sit in the seat of judgment that is reserved for God alone. Jesus instructs us to put down the stones we desire to throw, to put them down and take upon ourselves the mantle of Christ. In the AIDS epidemic it has been as if the people of the Church, hearing the words of Jesus, immediately picked up the largest stones they could find and hurled away. In the AIDS crisis church people have known the mandate to love our neighbor but have been distracted by the need to define human sin: differing sexuality, differing life-styles, drug abuse, and on and on. Thus distracted, the Church has been overtaken by the greatest sin of all: human hatred.

Most church people have tried to "sit this one out" because of AIDS identification with the gay estate, which many believe sinful. With few exceptions, church people have learned nothing from the epidemic, and yet we have had the chance to learn everything. The crisis presents us with the opportunity to learn again who we are, whose we are, and what we are to be about. The AIDS crisis calls us to look fearlessly at our identity as people of God.

I suspect our difficulty in seeing beyond the first blind spot results from our straying so far from a clear understanding of the meaning of the word *sin*. This has become one of society's buzzwords, despite the truth that *sin* has a very specific meaning. In earliest Aramaic and Hebrew, sin meant one thing: to miss the mark, to separate, to cause separation. Sin is that which separates us from ourselves, from our best view of ourselves, from each other, and it is that which separates us from our neighbor. Sin is that which divides a family, which separates us from wholeness. This is what sin has meant all along.

Sin is what we do knowingly or unknowingly. Sin is creating separation by casting out those we don't understand. Sin is what we say or fail to say. We all know this, but we forget.

Why? Because, my dear brothers and sisters, we love our separations, our distinctions—our safe distinctions. Our nature is indeed broken, flawed. We all know about Original Sin.

Religious fundamentalists of late dismiss Christ's imperative completely and set up as new graven images to be worshiped the very same levitical precepts and judgments that would stone to death anyone who breaks the puritanical, insistent, ritual-cleanliness code requirements. For those of us who have shaved, stoning is the penalty required by the codes. For a woman seen in public during her menstrual period, stoning is demanded. We do not find ourselves commanded to follow the levitical requirements of dietary, medicinal, architectural, or engineering practices of those days so long before Christ. We would not dream of hospitalizing our children within the medicinal compounds of those days. God forbid! Why in the name of God do we allow our society to be subjected to the dictates of the religious Right, which quotes those moralistic understandings as being the "last word" in the human/divine cooperative achievement? Our fundamentalist fellow Christians need to be challenged by the gospel and Jesus' new understanding. Jesus himself took on this same ruthless legalism. Challenging those defensive, exclusive ritual codes was exactly what got him nailed to the cross!

I call for an end to the caterwauling dictates of the theologically uneducated and undiscerning. Intelligent men and women, Christian and Jewish, in every community, must speak up and put an end to the religious Right's reign of hatred, judgmentalism, and bigotry.

The third blind spot is the sensitive issue of sexuality. Unfortunately, AIDS will probably always be known as a "gay" disease, despite clear evidence and heartbreaking statistics that heterosexuals by the thousands are afflicted in Africa and around the world, as well as here in the United States.

I believe we must address the misunderstanding, the bigotry, the judgmentalism involved in this area just as in every area where we deal with people we know little about. The levitical codes cited above are the source of Old Testament condemnation of homosexuality; however, we forget that condemnation is across-the-board for so many things we now understand differently. In addition to Leviticus, St. Paul is often quoted as homophobic justification. My beloved St. Paul; my ever-so-slightly judgmental Paul, to whom, I note, were we to convolute time, Christ did not entrust the keys of the Kingdom, perhaps seeing ahead to Paul's stoning of Steven. Our Lord entrusted those keys to the rougher, more expansively loving St. Peter. Paul reflects again and again the limited understanding of his day. While at times he rises out of his own humanity to heights of poetical brilliance, there are also embarrassing statements about the perpetuation of slavery, the second-class status of women, as well as his uneasiness about any area of human sexual expression.

Though he is respected and admired as the architect of early institutional Christianity, St. Paul is not the man any of us vowed to follow as our Lord and Saviour. The Christ, Jesus, the compassionate Lord of life and Lord of forgiveness and Lord of hope is the one we vowed to follow and by whom we shall ultimately be guided. We must tell that to our self-righteous, less-understanding brothers and sisters. We must stop being shy and say that clearly. If we do not, their souls will perish in the circle of misunderstanding and scorn they teach to so many as they club and scream their disdain for the outsider, the misunderstood, the different.

I believe that only now is the phenomenon of homosexuality becoming better understood, with new scientific insight, as one variation among many in the broad spectrum of human sexual expressions. Thinking clearly about this unselected estate and helping develop moral ideas within its expression would be far more appropriate for thinking Christian people than hurtling stones at those who, I assure you, have grown up to find this estate an unchangeable part of their existence.

Sadly, too many with AIDS wonder if there is any alternative but to go to the center of the circle and die.

Where are we in that circle? Where would Jesus be? Where would a saddened, loving St. Peter be? Where are you?

The roadblocks we have examined thus far are the toughest, yet from them we can emerge with insights that enable us to tackle a whole host of other social problems far more competently. The guide is simple and yet so hard.

We are to help our neighbor. Be brother to him. Sister to sister, a loving person to a loving person. As we move through our own fears and concerns and biases, we find the AIDS crisis invites us to view all of our experience with a rediscovered, clear, insightful, profoundly ethical, moral vision. This disease takes us into the very heart of darkness, human mean-spiritedness, to see how common that is to all the larger issues of society.

The fourth blind spot, concern for children in our society, is central to my anguish. I fear for them, for their culture is the great new arena of vulnerability. Kids, adolescents, have the same belief many of my gay friends had: that there are no consequences to sexual experimentation. Through such naiveté the human immunodeficiency virus, which has no orientation preference and is quite happy to be transmitted any way it can to whomever possible, runs rampant. When I look around me, the teenagers in our country today make up the only major group that believes there are no consequence to experimenting with sex. Statistics are beginning to confirm my worst fears for them and for those of you who are their parents.

Recently, at Grace Cathedral in San Francisco, I asked 150 parents and 50 teenagers how many teens in the room were having sex. Not a hand went up. When I met with the kids later without their parents, every hand in the room went up. When I asked if they were at least protecting themselves and their partners, again not a hand went up.

For heaven's sake, people, we need to get back to valid priorities: We need to get clear on the ethical priority that saving the lives of our kids is more important than saving our belief that they can somehow all magically abstain. Of course abstinence as our norm, our standard, is preferable for the sanctity of marriage and the long-honored commitments of sexual expression within that honorable institution, for our kids, as well as those called to marriage. But we need to be realistic. My experience with the decent young kids in that cathedral tells me that, if they are not all to die in the name of our traditional value system, we need to be realistic.

If condoms still are abhorrent in the face of common sense, then spray your kids head to foot in plastic. Get them educated. Get them protected. And very importantly, continue to teach that a long-time dedication of our bodies and hearts is infinitely to be preferred to the loneliness and heartbreak of one-night stands, the callousness and disillusionment that result and that can destroy the soul. The Church needs to take the lead in espousing these ethical priorities if our young folk are going to make it through this holocaust.

The Call of the Church

The AIDS crisis sounds a call to heal the ills of society: homophobia, hatred, bigotry, lack of moral values. In a society that has so many haves and have-nots, in a society that produces such despair and alienation and hopelessness in its poor that whole generations of young black, brown, yellow, and white people have drifted into drug abuse, prostitution, and crime, we must take the lead as Christian men and women to break the stranglehold those in power have on the powerless.

We must call for decent living standards for all people. Here in America that means looking more closely than ever before at those who lust for power, who would represent us in every level of government. How are dollars to be allocated? How much money for nuclear defense? How much money to feed, clothe, educate, raise up our broken? Oh, yes, we need to be in the business of setting moral standards. The gospel of Jesus empowers us, invites us, confronts us to do this, or else we shall all be overtaken by the despair and the shame and the brokenness, the complete societal destruction we are beginning to witness. If we are to treat AIDS, we must also treat the whole of our fractured society.

The Church, above all, should go on the line for the betterment of society. We must assemble our fold to reach out to not-so-safe places like the press and the government, calling for education, research, appropriate funding. We must advocate humane policies, while bringing the fold together to deal with complex data and real human need. The Church is called to initiate dialogue, to listen, to learn. We are called to the same unsettling journey as Abraham of old.

Above all the Church is called to be a moral guide for every age. We are called to start from traditional premises of morality, some good, some hateful, and examine and reexamine them critically and nondefensively to see which do conform to the mind and heart of Christ and which have strayed. We are called to seek new and ongoing guidance from the Holy Spirit. (One of our most pentecostal understandings is that the Holy Spirit asks us to change our views from time to time, although we dearly love to engrave them in stone and encyclical.) We are called to examine our positions to ascertain what is truly loving and needs growth, support, validation, and to be unafraid to view what has been hateful in our behavior and needs confessing and rewriting.

The Church needs to set an example for all who would truly look to her by apologizing for seeking the comfort of power and privilege. The time has come for the Church to repent her racism, her sexism, her anti-Semitism, as well as the homophobia she has fostered and taught and engraved in stone up through our time, contrary to Christ's imperative to understand and love and bind up.

I proclaim the gospel of Christ, which speaks for all the poor and powerless, the disenfranchised, the dispossessed who have died and who yet suffer from this disease; for abandoned black children; for kids denied education in many towns and cities; for young mothers dying alone; and for the sixty-seven gay friends I have lost.

While attempts to change are being made, some come too late. In the absence of the Church in the AIDS crisis, we who are dying have had to bear each other up alone, even to the very brink of our graves. We need the Church, all of us together as "struggling People of God" in the words of Hans Küng, to guide us in examining such issues as upholding the dignity of the little-understood, the different. We need to be loved, held, comforted—and enjoyed. We need to know that all humankind claim us as part of the gift of life. We need the Church to create guidelines, standards that take everyone's contemporary experience into account: men and women, not just the opinions of single male clerics, many of whom died hundreds of years ago.

Most of all, the Church needs to look beneath behavior to understand the underlying hopes and needs of people in their relationships, seen in the environments in which they live. The Church needs to understand the drives of people, what makes us tick, what makes us go on, what makes us hope, what enables us to survive with sanity and grace, as well as what crushes us into despair.

The Church needs to listen better and reflect more to try to understand us. For too long we have deliberated from a hierarchical, unquestioning mode. To listen and think, and to do both from the heart, is to become humane. Religions do not exist to make us religious. The role of religion is always to make us more humane. That is what it means to become brother-to-brother, sister-to-sister, neighbors to each other and thus to God who made us in all the infinite variations of his image and likeness.

God in the AIDS Crisis

Everywhere I turn I hear the cry, Where is God in this epidemic? Where is God in the sadness? Where is God in this human dilemma?

One day as a young curate, I was driving to my office. Teenagers in the car ahead of me deliberately sped up to hit a small crippled dog that had wandered in confusion onto the freeway. They hit it, and the dog flew up in the air to drop not far from where I was able to pull my car over. I got out, looking like a crazy man to those who saw me. I railed at God, "Where are you?"

When I got to my office, I took off my collar and threw it across the room, determined to give up and leave the ministry. Where was God?

A week had passed when in anguish I told my bishop, who with the wisdom of age and compassion looked at me and said, "God entered that situation when you stopped to pick up the animal and hold it while it died. In Mother Theresa's words of today, the dog was to know compassion and love as part of its experience in this life. God entered when you cared."

Whose hands but human hands? "For Mercy has a human heart, Pity a human face," wrote William Blake. In every tragedy like the crippled dog, like AIDS, like the ones you personally have faced, God comes into the circle when we bring him and the Divine light into it, when we stand up to show forth that love which is God. God comes into the tragedy when we respond to that challenge, when our compassion and clarity take on all that they must. The powers of evil are very great, and silence is its voice. A world is redeemed when Christ stands up and when we who would follow bearing his cross, his light, stand up, too.

I write to you as a churchman, your brother, a person with AIDS. I write as a man who regrets nothing of the love and goodness he has known, who stops now to notice flowers, children at play. I believe, to paraphrase St. Paul, that we are living, yet behold we die. Dying, behold we live. For I am persuaded that nothing can separate us from the love of God, neither height nor depth nor darkness nor despair—nothing can separate us from the love of God, if we love him and follow his commandment not to separate from each other and our compassion for each other.

For all of us as Church, I say to the world, "Help us! Join us!"

To you as Church, in a world that too often seems to prefer its darkness, I say from long-despairing peoples of all kinds, "Help us. Please help us. Be the gospel alive! Become what you are to become—grow into the potential God has willed for us."

For myself and those dying with me, in the long goodbye that is AIDS, I ask you not to forget us but to remember us sometimes and to surround us with your prayers, which you so mightily can do. Bear us up. For in all of our goodbyes and our looking back at so much that is stunning and dazzling and touching and truly important and valuable in life, I say, "Thank you, God. We bless you for our lives, for having raised us up from dust to know life and hope and the whole spectrum of what it is to be human. Thank you, God, for all our lives. Thank you. Give us courage to relinquish them with grace when it is time and give us hope for your Kingdom already breaking in upon each of us, even now. Thank you, God."

From Psalm 46, as paraphrased by Martin Luther:

> Let goods and kindred go,
> This mortal life also;
> The body they may kill:
> God's truth abideth still,
> His Kingdom is forever.

Biographical Note

William Barcus is on the staff of the Bishop of California, charged with overseeing the ministry of the church to persons with AIDS. Prior to that appointment he was executive director of the Episcopal Sanctuary, providing shelter for the homeless. He has served two congregations in San Francisco and one in Illinois. Before entering the Episcopal Theological School in Cambridge, he was in business.

The Violated Stranger

Mwalimu Imara

The essay by William Barcus is a statement about death in the midst of life, the death that crowds us when we violate the prime directive of love for the stranger who stands within our gates and when we are the violated stranger. The mood of his essay took me back to the fifties, when I responded to the rampant, oppressive racism that I first experienced as a new resident in this country. It scraped yesterday's fresh wound when my personhood was insulted and rejected for the hundredth—thousandth?—time by a presumptuous white man.

Cruelty and Hate

I see myself in Barcus's parable of the foxes. I have seen young black men killed in the street, beaten by men of the law for insisting on their right to vote and to move about as "free men" should. I have seen black women abused as they scrubbed the floors of the rich. I have seen black children in ghetto schools called stupid for asking questions. I have seen white society pound the life out of black people like the Holmes County foxes. I have seen hate and cruelty based on color, just as Barcus has seen hate and cruelty based on sex orientation.[1]

I have seen and felt the hate for my oppressors that came out of a thousand frustrations, daily abuses, and vilifications. I have felt the thick dryness in my throat and the hot acid in my stomach that came from a rage I dared not express for fear of my life and the safety of my children. I have grown tired of running, tired of holding my peace and guarding my tongue.

Preaching and moral exhortation do not get rid of hate. People hate in church as they do everywhere else. Hate is a built-in component of the kind of relationships that are judgmental, oppressive, authoritarian, racist, sexist, and heterosexist; but most especially hate is a component in relations between the weak and the strong, the haves and the have-nots, the chosen and the despised, the favored and the disinherited. Hate comes out of the systemic violence of the master/slave paradigm. The Church has

15

usually been on the side of the master. Seldom do we hear the Church address itself to the problems of those who have their backs against the wall.

Can the Church save us? Christ can. The Church might if it reaches behind Paul to Jesus. We often forget that Paul was a Jew and a free Roman citizen as well. Jesus was a Jew without the right of an appeal to the justice of Caesar. We forget that Jesus was a member of an oppressed people, and his good news offered a technique of survival for the oppressed. It was Jesus who pointed to the kingdom of God as being within us, giving oppressed people a ground to stand on that the fear and the domination of the oppressor could not take away.

> Once, having been asked by the Pharisees when the kingdom of God would come, Jesus replied, "The kingdom of God does not come visibly, nor will people say, 'Here it is,' or 'There it is,' because the kingdom of God is within you." (Luke 17:20, NIV)

Jesus gave to those whose backs were against the wall a place from which to reach out and grasp the power of God for a defense in the daily bombardment of injustice and fear.

From their pulpits, preachers should teach about the causes of hate and how it is generated by contact without fellowship among people. Too often they find it easier to sentimentalize and be comfortable on Sunday mornings.

Sanctuary

Canon Barcus reiterates the divine summons of the Church to the task of shepherding and providing sanctuary for those who are suffering and dying. The responses of the Church to this call are so labored, so minimal, and so late; that is the way of bureaucracies.

Years ago when I worked with terminally ill cancer patients and was trying to make hospice programs work for their families, I dreamed that the Church could do more to help us. Then the notion took hold of me that maybe, just maybe, hospice *was* the Church. The Church then became to me the heart, the mind, the endless labor of love and support given unstintingly to the dying and their families. This was the Church. As we worked to mend bodies and spirits, we felt the Holy Spirit in our midst. I have felt God as I witnessed for those in need who could not witness for themselves. I have been reinforced by the Spirit in a liturgy following a sacrifice of work in the quiet places or the marching witness of social protest. I guess I have come to expect no more than what the structure we call "the Church" gives, and I find myself surprised when it goes beyond these modest expectations. Perhaps I am just a cynic, but a cyclical cynic; when I mount up my next righteous charge I will be right out there in the halls of ecclesia demanding a programmatic response from the structure. My faith rests on the "still small voice."

Cynic or not, I guess the only sanctuary I know is in the hearts of people who make a welcome place for me that does not require me to be anyone except myself. These places are rare in my experience; they exist only in someone's caring. Sometimes that place is family; sometimes it is friends; sometimes it is both. Often that place is a hospice and occasionally a parish church. For me this is where God resides; this is my sanctuary. Each of us, if we would transform the Church, must become sanctuary for each other.

Blind Spots

In "our AIDS-generated blind spots" to which Barcus refers, the main thrust seems to deal with the judgment of homosexuality as being sinful. As a black person who is not gay, where do I begin to make common a ground between my perspective and Barcus' perspective as a person suffering from AIDS, a ground from which to reflect and respond?

Barcus begins with the problem of Christian arrogance and the consequent judgmentalism in addressing homophobia. My approach to the problems of racism and bigotry begins at another place. I cannot appeal only to the Christian Church for an end to racial injustice. The problem of black oppression is systemic in Euro-American societies. When I think of racism, I think of violence, specifically, structural violence.

> Structural violence is the most lethal form of violence because it is the least discernible; it causes premature death in the largest number of persons; and it presents itself as the natural order of things. A situation of oppression rests primarily on structural violence which in turn fosters institutional, interpersonal, and intrapersonal violence. Structural violence pervades the prevailing values, the environment, social relations, and individual psyches. The most visible indicators of structural violence are dif-

ferential rates of mortality, morbidity, and incarceration in the same society. In particular, a situation of oppression increases the infant mortality rate and lowers the life expectancy for the oppressed. Disparity on these dimensions is greater the more intense the socio-economic and structural violence.[2]

When I address American racism I see black men dying in numbers and at rates from all causes greater than any other group in the world. Black women and children follow closely, regardless of social status. When I relate to other liberation struggles, the magnitude of my black experiences overshadows and engulfs all dimensions of my concern. For instance, the careless injection with drugs is the principle mode of AIDS transmission in the black community, while transmission through unsafe sexual practices is the prime concern of the gay community. These two communities will have differing agenda as we struggle together against the same threats.

I have lent considerable energies to the women's struggle, but as white women move up the ladders of power to join their male counterparts they seem to be interested only in getting a bigger piece of the tainted pie; they have done little to lessen the death struggle of black people. Should we expect a different response for those struggling for recognition of differing life-styles? Gay white males and females are part of the system that maintains the oppression of my people, gay and straight. That does not mean that I will not support their struggle for liberation; I will. The evil of systemic oppression generalizes. Oppression cannot be kept isolated and must be fought wherever it surfaces. However, my expectations for reciprocation are modest. Experience again teaches black people to be cautious about alliances, even holy ones.

I support Barcus' definition of sin, and I believe we are on high ground. A basic spiritual issue for black people in the experience of racism is the way it destroys one's senses of personal dignity and integrity. We have to keep asking, "Who am I? What am I?" I imagine this is as true for the homosexual person in the process of self-discovery as in the experience of black people. To have to ask constantly whether or not "I belong" is to experience sin. Humans become human in dialogue with other humans. This process occurs in the family and is the model Jesus left us for the Church. To grow up feeling whole in situations that constantly challenge one's core identity is difficult. What did it do to my children to see me in situations with white people in which I was constantly threatened and without defense? What does it do to the psyche to be so vulnerable at such an early age?

I say "right on!" to Barcus's moral outrage at the pharisaic theology purveyed by the men and women of religion. Good "Christian America" sees blacks as immoral and violent without looking at the systemic immorality that creates those conditions. Steve Biko, the martyred South African black youth leader, wrote,

> Because the white missionary describes black people as thieves, lazy, sex-hungry, etc., and because he equated all that was valuable with whiteness, our Churches through our ministers see all these vices I have mentioned above not as manifestations of the cruelty and injustice which we are subjected to by the white man but inevitable proof that after all the white man was right when he described us as savages. Thus if Christianity in its *introduction* was corrupted by the inclusion of aspects which made it the ideal religion for the *colonization* of people, nowadays in its *interpretation* it is the ideal religion for the mainte-nance of the subjugation of the same people.[3]

Just as the Church has played a role as an oppressor and slave-maker, I remind myself that at the Church's core is the gospel that has been an effective manual for humane revolution. When I hear that I am a child of God and that the Kingdom of God is in me, I can buy some of Martin Luther King's courage in Christ and feel no fear from any person. When I get tired, impatient, and disillusioned with everyone, including myself, I can go to the same Bible that Harriet Tubman used for strength when she ran her freedom railroad. We struggle with the meaning of Christian ministry as Jesus himself defined it:

> The Spirit of the Lord is on me,
>   therefore he has anointed me
>   to preach good news to the poor.
> He has sent me to proclaim freedom for the prisoners
>   and recovery of sight for the blind,
> to release the oppressed,
>   to proclaim the year of the Lord's favor.
>
>   (Luke 4:18, 19, NIV)

Where Is God in the AIDS Crisis?

Barcus answered his own question of where is God in the AIDS crisis:

> I write to you as a churchman, your brother, a person with AIDS. I write as a man who regrets nothing of the love and goodness he has known, who stops now to notice flowers, children at play. I believe . . . that we are living, yet behold we die. Dying, behold we live. For I am persuaded that nothing can separate us from the love of God . . . if we love him and follow his commandment not to separate from each other and our compassion for each other.[4]

Our hearts are the locus for God in this crisis. Barcus lives with AIDS and suffers with its ravages and still loves us enough to take time out from what demands ultimate attention—his pain—to remind us, to encourage us to care and love, and to make our hands and hearts agents of the mission of God.

As the world shrinks, God is calling us to respond to the Holy Spirit and allow the material of the old world to go in order that God may create a new one. We will not begin to heal, learn from, and move beyond the holocausts of AIDS, hunger, drugs, exposure, and homelessness unless we turn from our materialistic, paternalistic, individualistic, self-gratifying, independent, competitive, rigid, over-rational, controlling, self-seeking living systems and replace them with humane values, becoming an inclusive, mutually affirming, interdependent, difference-appreciating, warm, cooperative, life-oriented, collectively responsible, self-questioning, God-seeking community. The gospel calls us to tear down the old way and build up the new, shingle by shingle, act by act, person by person, beginning with me.

References

1. So much of my theological thinking has been given shape by the ideas of Howard Thurman that I feel that I should footnote him whenever I articulate one of his many seminal themes. One such theme deals with Christianity as a religion for people who have their backs against the wall. This section was heavily influenced by his book *Jesus and the Disinherited* (Nashville: Abingdon Press, 1949).
2. H. A. Bulhan, *Frantz Fanon and the Psychology of Oppres-*

sion (New York: Plenum Publishing, 1985), p. 155.
3. S. Biko, *I Write What I Like* (San Francisco: Harper & Row, 1986), p. 57.
4. See preceding chapter.

Biographical Note

Mwalimu Imara is professor of medical ethics at the More-house School of Medicine in Atlanta. He is a graduate of Case Western Reserve University and earned a doctorate at the University of Chicago. He was associated with Elisabeth Kubler-Ross in Chicago and has written on the subject of death, dying, and the theology of hospice care.

Part 2.
The Clean and the Unclean

Introduction: The Clean and the Unclean

The nature of a human being is to seek out people who reinforce one's own sense of self. I enjoy the company of those who share my preferences in food, in music, in automobiles, in liturgical styles—those who have the good sense to have tastes similar to my own. We tend to cluster in groups, and each group, by the fact of its existence, excludes everyone else inhabiting the planet. This exclusive in-group alignment leads to moral judgments of worthiness/unworthiness, good/bad, guilty/innocent, and so on. We instinctively seem to establish we/they dichotomies in the social arena.

In the holocaust of AIDS, even the most conscious among us tend to do that. A dear friend, as open, accepting, and nonjudgmental as anyone I know, told me recently she is considering becoming a foster parent for an infant (or infants) born with human immunodeficiency virus (HIV). She went on to comment how innocent such infants are—they didn't do anything to deserve that. Her statements implied that noninfants so infected were not innocent and as members of the out-group were deserving of their fate.

In the extemporaneous discussion at the conference, Patricia Wilson-Kastner responds to this human dilemma by describing the challenge to the Church: "We are called upon to seriously grapple, in worship and in word, with what it means to be an inclusive community, with a God who calls all people in grace, and calls us all to live together in the same church in the same field at the same time, standing right next to each other."

The estrangement created by exclusionary attitudes and the resulting hostility of the excluded pose a grave challenge to Christians who wish to respond to the call of God to be an inclusive community. As William Countryman explains, "Much of the repugnance many Christians have toward dealing with AIDS derives from their repugnance for homosexuality. The questions about sexual ethics become very important, and the questions about the pure and the impure in that particular vein become very important. The Church lost the right sometime

25

back, several centuries at the very least, to have very much of a role in discussing with gay and lesbian people the issue of sexual ethics, just as the Church lost the right a long time back to participate with Jews in an analysis of the meaning of the Holocaust. We may at times be tolerated in that discussion, but we don't have a right to enter into it. It is a topic we must handle with some delicacy."

Frightening Grace

The life of grace offers a freedom many of us find frightening. Our anxieties are provoked by life in a pluralistic society where our convictions about "the right" and our need for "order" result in fearfulness because they are not reinforced by the chaotic pluralism that is our world. Wilson-Kastner speaks with intentional irony to these fears: "In our relationship to God and the Church what we would really like to do for our security is to impose what we know to be 'the right' on the world so that things may be 'in order' and we can be 'in control'; that means there have got to be objective standards of morality which 'we know' and 'we tell people to do.' These things are of course self-evident to us and because they are self-evident to us it is what ought to govern the world. [People have] an enormously strong tendency . . . to impose this kind of ethics on the world and, if they can, [to also] impose their standards [of] 'what God wants.' We [often] have not offered any kind of alternative. . . . [We have failed to challenge them to have a] living relationship to God! [As a result of that failure], the positive part of their religion is following certain laws. [They believe] 'that's what religion is about!' [For them] God is the one who says, 'That's what you ought to do, and I will reward you here or later, depending upon the system you follow.' [We often speak] of having a relation with God as the center of [one's] religion, and having the Church as a community of believers. We use [these] phrases but I think [they] are really quite empty in most people's experience. I think that we are not only wrestling with the question of how to talk about ethics but we are wrestling with it in the context of a community in which people have nothing else to put in place of a rigid, judgmental ethical approach."

Is God's Love Enough?

Is simply asserting that God loves us sufficient? How can we know what God expects of us? The Bible, in places such as the Book of Hebrews, speaks of purity issues, and in the *Book of Common Prayer* the Ash Wednesday service refers to our "self-indulgent appetites and ways," our envy, our "intemperate love of worldly goods," our "waste and pollution of your creation." Edward Franks, of the presiding bishop's staff, raises the question, "What constitutes an acceptable state in the eyes of God other than the fact that God loves us?"

Purity, according to Countryman, is not the only virtue, and impurity is not the only sin. The New Testament rejects the notion of purity [that we read of in the Hebrew scriptures] related to the Temple and to the purity laws of Leviticus, [along with] the notion that [such purity] is what grants access to God. If it does, the Gentiles are totally out of luck. The New Testament rejects that notion. It sets in its place a metaphorical purity of the heart. Purity of the heart is concerned with not harming your neighbor, not taking what belongs to your neighbor, not doing any evil to your neighbor. That kind of purity is still a part of Christian behavior, for the New Testament. I think the two have to be clearly distinguished from each other. On one level the New Testament is saying, 'Salvation is not limited by being Jewish, it's not limited by being pure, because salvation is through the cross of Christ and not through the Temple.' Then there is something much deeper than that going on, which says that salvation is not even by righteousness, or at least not by our righteousness. It is by forgiveness."

The theology of grace of Augustine of Hippo is an area of special study for Wilson-Kastner. "For Augustine, grace does not consist of God's ignoring our evil but in the transformation of the whole person through the indwelling of the Holy Spirit. . . . Even though person A, who does not have the indwelling of the Holy Spirit, and person B, who does, may do the same things, one is virtuous because it comes from the Holy Spirit within; the other does the same wonderful things but isn't virtuous."

Students of religion and sexuality are aware that Augustine had perhaps the most radically dualistic view of the body of any of the church fathers and was implacably hostile toward sexual feelings. Wilson-Kastner refers to this saying, "Augustine has enormous difficulty imagining how one can correlate human sexuality with the indwelling of the Holy Spirit. He finds it really hard to talk about sexual ethics, except by ultimately excluding as much sex as possible. That means our heritage is in real trouble! One of the things we have to factor in is that we do in fact have traditions which don't know how to put together these different strands of the Scripture. Some [traditions] want to live in the Old Testament and have laws which say what is pure and what is impure; others have grasped the New Testament insight of the heart-relationship to God, [as well as a heart-relationship] to others. [That will then become] the norm through which we talk about ethical behavior. But we haven't even seriously explored the difficulty together, much less developed a vocabulary in context within which to talk about Christian response and behavior."

God and Nature

The institutional church, in some times and places, has been highly exclusionary on the basis of sexual orientation and skin color, often appealing to theology, specifically a theology of natural law. Randy Frew, of the Presiding Bishop's staff, raises the issue in quoting those who assert that God the Creator made "Adam and Eve, not Adam and Steve." Those churches have held that "persons of color are not as genuine as persons who are Caucasian. . . . What will happen to the next generation of persons with AIDS because they are already hated because of their color?"

Frederick Borsch reminds us that the Church didn't invent homophobia and racism and that often people who cite natural theology to support their views are not church members. "It exists quite strongly outside the Church," and in many cases they didn't learn it from the Church. "The Church has had a role in trying to overcome these things in the life of society."

The church community can work toward overcoming the horrors of homophobia and racism through two kinds of activities, states Wilson-Kastner. "I think we all need to be much clearer and more mature and developed about what we do affirm as Christians, what kind of relationship with God we affirm: a relationship which is worth living and dying for. Frankly, in most of the preaching I have heard, from others and from myself, the quantity of passionate love of God and neighbor which is involved would fill a teeny little bit of a small styrofoam cup. We often have so little to offer people it is no wonder that what is in their hearts and souls gets filled up with all this [bigotry] from the culture, which has been in it since Adam and Eve and Steve all evolved. We need to offer people a strong, mature relationship with God.

"Another kind of thing we need to do in our counseling, our preaching, our conversations, our visitations as clergy and laity, our Christian education committees [is] a constant bird-dogging of issues. Those snide comments that come up at coffee hour; those questions about where should we send our money in the benevolence committees; [those questions about] what kind of program should we have for Christian education and about sexuality, abortion, racism, our domination by the middle-class perspective (What about the folks who aren't middle class?)—what about all those things that go on? It is very tiring, but absolutely essential, that week after week, month after month, year after year, we persist in helping people come to terms, in small and big ways, with what hate, anger, fear, frustration, animosity, and persecution of other people do and what the gospel offers us as an alternative. It involves persistence.

"Jonathan Edwards said that the difference between false enthusiasm and true conversion is persistence. True conversion is persistent, through one's whole life. Part of the reality of what we face is we are not talking about two weeks of intense work with AIDS; we are talking about our lives as individuals and as a church. We need to be prepared for the work of a lifetime."

Bumper-Sticker Theology

Many of the attitudes toward people of different races and sexual orientations that prevail in the United States have been reduced to slogans. Countryman reminds us that throughout history people have used theological slogans, and as lamentable as that might be, perhaps we can respond with slogans. He proposes that the question that must be asked of all Christians— liberals, evangelicals, and fundamentalists alike—must be, Where is the good news? You call this evangel; you call this gospel. Where is the good news for anybody who doesn't happen to be just like you to start with? Sermons in the Episcopal Church are not usually about the good news. They may be about the gospel for the day, but they are not usually about the good news. They are usually refinements of some theological theme or theme of concern for the parish. They are sometimes law of another kind, insisting that you agree with this scheme rather than the evangelical scheme.

"If we are going to insist on the good news we must be sure we know what we are talking about when we call it good news. I find when I press seminarians on the subject they can't give me an account of what they understand to be the good news. I can't blame them for that because I'm not sure I could have four or five years ago either, because nobody had ever asked me in the Episcopal Church! I had no need for the knowledge! I think we need the knowledge now."

Tell Me the Old, Old Story

People begin to understand the meaning of a personal relationship with God and to experience the good news of which Countryman speaks, when they encounter authentic compassion in the context of human relationship. As William Doubleday states, whether "we talk about the AIDS issue or the gay issue or the intravenous drug abuse issue or the race issue, relationships with people, [the opportunity] to know somebody who is different from ourselves, who lives in that category which we previously excluded, is in fact [the process of] converting and transforming in a profoundly evangelistic sense." Doubleday, who has been on the "AIDS lecture circuit" for several years, recounts that frequently, after hearing human stories of real people, listeners would come to him and confess, "I'm going to invite my son to come home after all" or "I'm going to call my brother whom I haven't talked to for twenty years."

Doubleday sees the experience of listening to stories, rather than being confronted with Scripture or theological rhetoric, as "a kind of conversion, the same kind of conversion that gay people, recovering alcoholics, and recovering drug abusers also go through in terms of their own process of coming to a more positive sense of who they are in relationship to God." The "right theology" doesn't have nearly the likelihood of developing a real relationship with God as does the face-to-face relationship with an individual living in a category that one previously excluded.

Doubleday urges us to continue "to talk about who Jesus related to. The ministry of compassion, the ministry of healing of Jesus Christ transcended categories; in fact, it broke into categories which were clearly unclean, taboo outcasts. That kind of paradigm can inform all of us in pastoral care."

Sinning Away the Holy Spirit

Frequently talking about the gospel may evoke persecution, Countryman asserts, particularly when we speak to people who are resisting the good news. We must speak with people who disagree with us out of our own experience, when our feet are "on the ground." "In the process we will encounter the one group of people whom the gospel cannot reach, who are committing the sin against the Holy Spirit. It is usually religious people, the Pharisees in the Gospel, and it's religious Christians amongst us. The sin against the Holy Spirit is looking at a good act which gives hope and life to someone and saying, 'That's evil because it wasn't done by my group and it isn't consistent with my theology.' It is the person who can say to you, 'That's not love because it is between two men or two women and doesn't fit my definitions,' who is committing that sin. We cannot help that person except by witnessing to what has happened to us."

"Ultimately, anything that really matters comes out of personal relationship," according to Wilson-Kastner. "We have to be prepared with all the cognitive arguments, and we also have to remember personal and social relations—they are all interconnected. We speak with mind and heart and spirit and offer people [our] experience. We do not understand concepts, but we relate to people and [then they] begin to understand and articulate cognitively. It is the heart which moves first."

"People are afraid," Borsch observes. "People are full of fear. Life is a very insecure business. People are grasping to know what group they belong to and for some kind of security. The louder people bluster, the more I figure they are afraid. Unless we can offer them security, a sense of love and being cared for, I don't think we are ever going to get very far—and that's what the gospel has to offer. Unless we can reach out to them with some experience of healing and love and compassion in our own lives, they are not going to be changed by any of our arguments. Our task, always, is to convince them that 'I really care for you (even though you are the most bigoted person I ever met!) because God cares for you and I care for you.' Then I think we can have some kind of meeting. That is the central concern which must run through all of our pastoral care."

Rosa Escobar: I am coming from the San Juan Bautista Episcopal Church in the South Bronx. I would like to bring a little something that happened to me this week. I was coming to my job, and I found a lady that I know in the street, and she told me, "Mrs. Escobar, are you working in the Episcopal Church?" And I say, "Yes." And she told me, "Can you come to me to the hospital?" And I answered, "What happened?" And she say, "Well, you know, my husband is in the hospital." And I answered, "What happened to him?" And she told me, "He's with AIDS." That very moment I told her, "I go with you to the hospital." And she told me, "Can you go by yourself and ask for him because I have to stay home and take care of my children?"

So I went to the only hospital we have in the South Bronx, to the Lincoln Hospital. I went to the information, and I asked, "Is Mr. José Rios here?" And she told me, "Well, lady, I have to look in the machine." She went to the machine, and she told me, "No, is no one by that name here." And I told her, "I'm sure he's here because I just talked to his wife and she told me he is here." And she told me, "Let me check on information." She went to the machine, she checked on information, and he wasn't there. But I don't give up. I start to walk around in emergency room, and I saw this door that say, "Do Not Enter. Contagious Diseases." And I say to myself, "Well, maybe he is there!" And I look all over to see if I saw I police; I don't saw anyone, so I pushed the door. Sure it was. The man was there. The IV he was supposed to have was dry to the limit. His lip was bleeding. That man was there for three days, and nobody cares. And that is the situation we have in our communities, in the black and Hispanic communities. It's not only gays; it's gays, black, and Hispanic.

We Have Met the Church and It Is Us

The lapel pin distributed at the Episcopal General Convention in the summer of 1988 read, "Our Church Has AIDS." Wilson-Kastner describes the difficulties we are facing in the Church as both a wonderful opportunity and a challenge. "We are trying now, consciously and unconsciously, to admit who we are. Over the last couple of thousand years we have pretended that the

Church is the able-bodied heterosexual [Anglo-Saxon] male who writes the prayers and governs the church. Everybody else is somebody we pray for or do good to. Note the words of the intercessions: 'Let us pray for the aged, the infirm, the hoo hoo and the wat wat.' Most of the Church *is* the aged and the infirm! What are we talking about?

"Now, I am not being entirely facetious. The Church *is* gay people. It is not ministering to gay people; they are us; we are us. The Church is Hispanic. It is poor, of various races. The Church is a whole lot of people who, somehow, we haven't quite made part of the self-awareness and the articulation of the Church's identity and sense of communion.

"One of the things we are struggling with and need to struggle with is who are we? And how can we talk to each other and listen to each other, with our multiplicity of experiences and backgrounds, in such a way that we respect each other as members of the Body of Christ and try to be mutually helping and loving to each other, not on my terms, but in terms of the common good? I think we are reaching new, painful stages of awareness of what this might mean and [what the] challenges [are] to us. I think it is difficult, painful, and hopeful. I hope that part of what we will do is continue with that work of self-awareness and respect for one another."

For the Clean or the Unclean?

Louis William Countryman

In the still relatively short history of the AIDS crisis, the Christian churches have occupied an equivocal position. Christians have been in the forefront of compassionate response and also have determinedly lagged behind. The churches have encouraged education about safe sexual practices to prevent the further spread of the disease, and they have also resisted any open discussion. Old enmities with gay and lesbian people have been cast aside in the name of a common concern for the sick, and these enmities also have been exacerbated by calling AIDS a divine judgment on people whom the church has rejected. The picture is very perplexing and muddled.

In part, these differences are between one denomination and another—not altogether surprising, given our enormous diversity. In part, the differences are between one faction and another within a given denomination, for in every community members are prone to emphasize different values within the common tradition. In part, the differences arise from the contrasting experience of congregations. The urban parish that has first cared for and then buried many of its most devout and faithful members will see the matter rather differently from a suburban or small-town parish that has not been touched by the disease or that, as sometimes happens, refuses to acknowledge that the disease has touched any church member.

Yet something more is at work here than simple differences of tradition or of interpretation or even of personal experience. I think that in most, perhaps all, of us the ambiguity and uncertainty goes far deeper, so that whatever our tradition and experience may be, we feel pulled in more than one direction. There is indeed a division within the Christian message, as it has long been proclaimed, that creates division within us as individuals and communities. Hence the odd spectacle of the Church trying to be in the vanguard and the rear guard at the same time.

If this is true, then we must return, here at the beginning of this discussion, to the most fundamental aspects of our Christian faith in order to understand who we really are as people of the gospel. Not only for our own sakes do we need to do this—so that we may know our own mind and the mind of the gospel in this matter. It is also for the sake of those whom we serve: people with AIDS, their families, partners, and friends; those irrationally terrified of AIDS, those exposed to it, with or without understanding their danger; children who must grow up in its presence; and even those who are trying to ignore the whole matter. We cannot address or serve others in a straightforward and appropriate manner so long as we are uncertain about the promise and power of the gospel on which we rely and from which our ministry stems.

This exploration may be helped if we begin by looking at what pulls us toward and away from a particular role in relation to the AIDS crisis. Then we can look at the way in which these influences are comparable to those that affected Christians at other critical moments in our history and how these influences reflect the deepest issues of our faith.

Christians are drawn to an active role in the AIDS crisis by our long tradition of service to all in need. This, of course, goes back to Jesus, both in his example as healer and washer of feet and in his teachings. "The son of humanity did not come to be served but to serve and to give his life as ransom for many" (Mark 10:45). The needs occasioned by AIDS are obvious and do not require any further documentation here. Yet what is often overlooked in discussing the problem in the United States is that the crisis particularly affects people relegated to the margins of Western society. The Church has long felt particular responsibility toward just such persons. In the United States the rates of infection among blacks and Hispanics are substantially higher than for the white population; in the world at large the troubles of this country are a drop in the bucket compared to what threatens some central and eastern African nations. There, according to one knowledgable friend of mine, an entire generation of young, educated people may well be wiped out, with dismal consequences for the countries that have invested so much treasure and hope in them. The Church is not a national organization but a world community. If we are not aware of the global scope of the crisis, who will be? The great needs confronting us, here and abroad, are more than enough to call forth the Christian response of service, whether in the area of education or in care for the sick, dying, and bereaved.

For another reason, Christians are becoming involved in ministry specifically to persons with AIDS and their loved ones. AIDS has once again brought death into the midst of life in a way that seemed almost unthinkable in the United States just a few years ago. Our secular culture is terrified of death, but for Christians death is not an end but a transition. We believe in the God who brought Jesus our shepherd from the dead, and we therefore expect to find in death an illumination of life and faith. Francis of Assisi is not the only saint to have celebrated Sister Death or to have found a ministry among those near to her. If we, too, find ourselves owing reverence and service to the dying, this is not because of some morbid fascination with death. Still less should we desire to impose our own piety on people weakened by sickness. Rather, we recognize that the God of the resurrection is met in a new way at the gate of death and that every death is a sacred act, whatever the particular circumstances.

Still other considerations pull Christian people back from active service in this crisis. Most important among these is that at first the disease in the United States was largely confined to two groups that many Christians have traditionally defined as immoral: homosexual men and intravenous (IV) drug abusers. Of these, the churches have been, I think, less critical of the drug abusers, perhaps because the experience of Alcoholics Anonymous has alerted us to the complexities of addiction. Then, too, IV drug abusers do not form a coherent or highly visible group within most Christian churches; this has made them easier for us to ignore. Gay and lesbian people, on the other hand, were actively engaged in coming out of the closet and seeking full status in the Church when the AIDS crisis began. The argument over the moral status of their sexual orientation and their varieties of sexual behavior was already underway. For a great many Christians, this posed the question of whether ministry to people with AIDS would appear to be offering approval to people whose sexual orientation and manner of life they regard as seriously immoral.

Like the tradition of Christian service, this concern for defining and maintaining moral standards has very old roots in Christianity, stretching back to the New Testament itself. At a very early time we find Paul telling the Christians at Corinth to shun church members who were leading seriously immoral lives (1 Cor. 5:9–13). The later New Testament epistles continued and perhaps intensified this theme, demanding of every Christian the highest possible moral standards. Their concern was partly based on anxiety about maintaining a good reputation among non-Christian neighbors, an important consideration in a time of threatened or actual persecution (e.g., 1 Pet. 2:11–12). However, this also continued a long-standing concern of religious Jews to preserve themselves and their religion by a distinctiveness that would mark them off from the world around them. In this respect, the early Christians were carrying on an ancient inheritance, as are their modern successors who speak of having to "draw the line" or "hold the line somewhere." Communities and traditions have to have shape, and shape implies boundaries.

Two very different conceptions of Church confront each other here. One sees Church as a community that finds life in giving to outsiders; the other sees Church as a community that must define and maintain purity with great care. Ultimately, both conceptions may be necessary; yet, opposite as they are, they cannot coexist as equals. One or the other must have the final word. One or the other must serve as the touchstone by which the reality of Christian life and faith will be revealed. For whom, then, does the Church exist? For the insiders or for the outsiders? For the pure or for the impure? For the righteous or for sinners? These are questions, not only about the nature of the Church, but about the nature of the gospel, the good news, that gave rise to the Church. They are questions that stand at the very heart of our faith.

There is a longstanding tradition, of course, that the Church is the company of the pure—or the relatively pure. This tradition is rooted in the experience of Israel, a nation set apart, called to be the peculiar possession of its God. At the heart of this nation, according to the Torah, was God's sanctuary—at first the Tent of Meeting, in later years the Temple of Jerusalem. No unclean thing might enter into this sanctuary. Priests must be free of any personal blemish or handicap, and, as women are more prone to uncleanness as defined by the Torah, priests must be male. The sacrificial animals must be those defined as clean for human consumption, and each individual animal must be free of blemishes.

The sanctuary was the center of purity, the place to be preserved with greatest care. All the people, however, were obligated to keep a degree of purity, in accordance with detailed instructions laid out, for the most part, in Leviticus. In Jesus' time, the most devout Jews, such as Essenes and Pharisees, sought to go beyond what the Torah required and observe the purity of the Temple in all its rigor even in their own homes or communities. This represented, of course, a very high degree of commitment to their religion, requiring constant effort and vigilance. In dedicating themselves to the goal of remaining as close as possible to God, as though they were living in the Temple itself, the Essenes and Pharisees represented an acme of piety and devotion seldom equalled since their time.

In its history, the Church has also had moments of great fervor in the pursuit of purity. In the fourth century, such Christians as Jerome extravagantly praised the religious value of virginity, and many committed themselves to a monastic life believed to be purer and more acceptable to God than that of the average Christian. The conviction that God is pleased by purity, defined primarily in the avoidance of things sexual, has remained part of Christianity ever since. This definition of purity differed from that of Leviticus but came to be dominant among Christians from about the fourth century onward. What remained from Leviticus was the conviction that purity, however defined, brings a person close to God. The classic English proverb, ''cleanliness is next to godliness,'' is a somewhat watered-down form. In reality most Christians have long believed that, in some sense, ''cleanliness,'' especially sexual purity, is at the heart of godliness.

This is not a New Testament teaching. Strictly speaking, it is not even biblical teaching. For Leviticus, purity is a category that reaches far beyond sexual issues and includes matters of food, agricultural practice, weaving, skin disease, worship, death, justice, kindness. Virginity was not a principal aspect of purity anywhere in the Bible, with the possible exception of Revelation, which at one point holds up a group of 144,000 male virgins (14:1–5) as an example or as a symbol whose meaning is now difficult to grasp. The intense emphasis on virginity arose during and just after the New Testament era and was originally associated with marginal teachers rejected by the mainstream of the Church (e.g., 1 Tim. 4:1–3).

Still, we must acknowledge that a concern for purity, however defined, is deeply rooted in our tradition. The Reformers, for example, when they rejected the idea that virginity is somehow superior to all other forms of Christian life, did not reject the value of purity but redefined purity in terms of married chastity and fidelity. Something tugs Christians very strongly to define ourselves in terms of purity. What is it? In part, of course, it is simply the tradition. We both read the Scriptures and inherit our basic outlook from our immediate forebearers in the Church; from these sources we imbibe a concern for purity. Still, all Christians, of whatever variety, have exercised great freedom in relation both to Scripture and to tradition. Leviticus is not widely read, and most modern church people would find Jerome's attack on marriage scandalous. Why, then, does purity remain important?

No doubt wanting to "hold the line somewhere"—that phrase that one hears so often in discussions related to AIDS and to gay and lesbian people—plays an important role. As we seek a sense of identity, we are seeking for boundaries—some tangible line that we can draw around ourselves and be quite sure who is on which side. Purity serves that boundary function well. To preserve purity means both to assert certain standards and to behave in certain objective ways. We are those who maintain the standards. People who disagree about the standards or violate them are easily identified as other than we.

This is the usefulness of purity—and also the source of the problems surrounding it. I have already noted that, in the time of Jesus, the Pharisees and Essenes were particularly committed to keeping purity. The Essenes are never mentioned in the Gospels, perhaps because they were rather reclusive. The Pharisees, however, appear often. In some respects, Jesus and the early Christians were closely related to them. Like the Pharisees, they believed in a resurrection of the dead at the last day. Like the Pharisees, and unlike the literalist Sadducees, they used the written Scriptures of Israel somewhat freely in the proclamation of their own interpretation of the faith; they were, so to speak, "liberals." In other respects, however, the earliest Christians were diametrically opposed to the Pharisees, not least in the matter of purity.

Jesus was criticized because he tolerated uncleanness in his disciples. Indeed, most of his disciples were quite ordinary Jews who were much less careful in such matters than Pharisees. One, we are told, was even a tax collector; they were always suspected of uncleanness, perhaps because they dealt with Gentiles and had to enter so many different houses and be exposed to so many sources of impurity. Once, at dinner in the house of a Pharisee, Jesus allowed a woman who was a notorious sinner to come up behind him as he reclined at table and touch him. He hardly can have supposed that she was meticulous about purity (Luke 7:36–50). On another occasion Jesus carried on a long conversation with a Samaritan woman of ill repute and even made her a missionary, despite his disciples' disapproval (John 4). A woman with a hemorrhage, which made her as impure as if she were menstruating and rendered her uncleanness contagious to others, touched Jesus as she sought a miracle of healing. He did not condemn her but sent her away whole and in peace (Mark 5:25–34). He himself, on more than one occasion, came into contact with dead bodies, a virulent source of impurity, in the process of raising people from the dead (Mark 5:41; Luke 7:14). In short, the Gospels present to us a Jesus who, for a Jewish religious teacher of the first century, was scandalously indifferent to the purity code incumbent on all Jews—still more so to the one insisted on by Pharisees.

Why did Jesus behave in this way? It may seem a small matter to us who scarcely know the levitical code and do not care about it. But we must understand that Jesus' behavior, in the context of his own day, made him appear radically unclean, unrespectable, and subversive of public morals. What purpose could such behavior possibly have for his ministry? It alienated the most religious and respectable people of the day, and this must have helped lead to his crucifixion. (It is always easier, after all, to inflict summary punishment on those who are not respectable.)

The answer may lie in the audience that Jesus was seeking out. According to Matthew (9:13), Jesus said, "I have not come to call the righteous, but sinners." (Luke 5:32 adds "to repentance," but that is not in Matthew, who almost certainly wrote before Luke.) He gathered his disciples, for the most part, from among the most ordinary of Jews, not the most religious. John tells us that he had a few followers among the religious authorities, but they remained closeted for fear of detection (19:38–39); the mass of Jesus' followers were more or less unclean from the perspective of the Pharisees. Jesus displayed a consistent preference for the company of "tax collectors and sinners," as the evangelists put it. On one occasion he even said to the religious authorities that the tax collectors and prostitutes were going into the Realm of the Heavens ahead of them (Matt. 21:31). If this does not make all of us good church people of the twentieth century a little nervous, it probably should!

What was Jesus driving at? He was deliberately transgressing the boundary that divided the clean from the unclean. Why? Perhaps the nature of the boundary itself had prompted his teaching and actions. In principle, purity existed as a way to draw near to God's holiness, something that gave access to the sanctuary. In practice, purity always becomes not a means to God but a means to self-aggrandizement and to scorn of neighbor. Jesus told a story about a Pharisee who went up to the Temple and thanked God that he was not like the tax collector he saw there, also praying. The Pharisee in this parable was not particularly malicious; the pure are always making comparisons between themselves and others. In the process, however, his own virtue became the central motif of his prayer, which thus degenerated into a gesture toward himself and his own goodness. The tax collector, on the other hand, could find no claim to make for himself and threw himself instead on God's mercy. He, says Jesus, went down to his house justified (Luke 18:9–14).

The point seems to be that the pure glorify themselves, while the impure are free to seek and glorify God. On the whole, Jesus probably observed the purity law of Israel in some fashion or other. Yet he insisted on breaking down the wall that that purity law erected, not only between Jew and Jew, but between Jew and Gentile also. According to Luke, Jesus praised the faith of a gentile centurion, an officer of the occupying army, as greater than any he had encountered in Israel itself (Luke 7:9). He admitted that a Greek-speaking woman (Matthew even calls her a Canaanite) had bested him in argument (Mark 7:24–30; Matt. 15:22). While his work was normally confined to the people of Israel, he began to break through this greatest of purity boundaries in his earthly ministry.

Even with Jesus' example before them, the early Christians had a hard time believing it was possible to step across purity boundaries. According to Luke, it took a direct revelation from God before Peter was willing to preach the good news to a gentile family, and the Holy Spirit had to fall upon the new converts in a highly manifest way before Peter thought of baptizing them

(Acts 10). The whole story of Acts is, to a great extent, the story of how Jewish Christians, maintaining their concern for some level of levitical purity, accommodated to the idea that Gentiles, seen as ritually unclean, could be Christians, too. Many, of course, were prepared to allow Gentiles to join the church provided they became Jews and adhered to Jewish standards of purity. The great question was whether a Gentile, particularly a male in all his uncircumcised uncleanness, could remain a Gentile and yet be a Christian. The answer, in due course, was yes. But the struggle was a long and sometimes bitter one. We modern Christians have no monopoly on churchly divisiveness.

The issue involved was and is a serious one. To have an identity, a religious community must have boundaries. Boundaries mean there will be outsiders. If the boundaries are those of purity, the religious will begin to look down on the irreligious, the clean on the unclean. The result is a piety no longer focused on God but on the pious, on their purity and virtue. Here is the nub of the thing. Jesus found himself in conflict with the Pharisees not because the Pharisees were bad people but because they were good people—very good people, eminently respectable. He did not find himself in conflict primarily with their thought or their principles but with their goodness and the self-confidence that it engendered.

God's good news of forgiveness, according to Jesus, overcomes all the distinctions that the religious draw between themselves and others. God understood that all are guilty, not just the egregiously impure. God has already forgiven all, not just the worthy or the relatively worthy; the nearly clean or the almost completely pure. God's act of grace is central, not the worthiness of the recipient. In the parable of the prodigal the father does not stand on his dignity or wait to hear a repentant speech from this son who has been off wallowing with the pigs. No, he runs out to meet him while he is still a long way off. Meantime the other son, the loyal, pious, dutiful one, complains that his brother has not deserved any of this, that his brother does not measure up to his own example (Luke 15:11–32). And that, of course, is just the point. The tax collectors and prostitutes enter the Reign of the Heavens ahead of the religious because they know how to rejoice in God's goodness while we, the religious, want God to appreciate our goodness.

Paul made the same point more methodically and, in the process, offered a kind of solution to the problem of where purity belongs in the Christian faith. Paul constantly emphasized the priority of God's grace over human works (e.g., Rom. 5:6–8). We do not and cannot save ourselves. Even the best of human beings (and Paul felt that he belonged in that class himself [Phil. 3:4–6]) find an abrupt and unexpected limit to their ability to understand and obey what God wills. This is why the Church could include Gentiles as easily as Jews—because neither group really had anything to claim on behalf of itself. Israel, to be sure, enjoyed the great gift of the Torah and the prophets, but this was precisely a gift, a grace. It was not to the credit of Israel that it enjoyed such things but to the credit of God who gave the gift to them. If the Jews were clean while the Gentiles were unclean, that was something for Jews to be thankful for and not to feel superior about.

God's grace is able to put anyone right—or "justify" anyone, as we traditionally say in English. Being put right, however, does not mean that you have to become clean in accordance with the laws of physical purity in Leviticus. If that were so, Gentile males would still have had to be circumcised, and, as Paul pointed out, those who were circumcised would then have been obligated to keep the entire Torah (Gal. 5:3). Better, then, for them to remain as they were and rely purely and solely on God's gifts. Paul, in fact, wanted all Christians, Jews and Gentiles, to remain as they were, for he feared that change in either direction would manifest some doubt of God's goodness and power, some sense that one would be better off if only one did thus and so (1 Cor. 7:17–20; Gal. 6:15).

To be better off than you are when you have just been saved by God's goodness is hardly possible. Why would anyone even think of such a thing? Sin prompts such a notion—and sin of the most serious kind: the sin of works-righteousness. To be recipients of a gift is a wonderful thing; but to be givers of gifts would, we think, be even better, or, at least to receive God's grace as our due rather than as an undeserved gift. The besetting sin of humanity, the desire to put ourselves in the place of God, emerges in this most corrupting form among the religious and is characteristic of all religious life. This is the sin of the prodigal's brother who does not want to admire God's goodness because he would rather have God admire his, the elder brother's, virtue.

Well, in that case, would not getting rid of religion and its corrupting effects altogether be better? No. For one thing, sin is not that easily fooled. We cannot defeat sin merely by abolishing one or another of its pretexts; human beings will still desire to play God and will find other venues in which to do it. For another thing, religion—specifically, the Church—serves a vital function. The Church may not proclaim the good news well; but without the Church who will proclaim it at all? Without the Church, where will we gather to hear the story of salvation, to be washed in baptism and fed with the Body and Blood of Christ, to encourage one another and to be encouraged, to have our hope renewed and to practice the love that is the hallmark of our new life? Religion is not dispensable; the Church is not dispensable. But we have to watch it like a hawk. Which is to say, we have to watch ourselves. We say that we want to tell the world about the goodness of God, but often we talk instead about our own goodness.

This is how the purity rules came back into the Church, I suppose, or rather how new ones were created within the Church. Only a few small Christian sects ever have returned to the actual purity code of Leviticus. Instead, what we have done is construct new purity systems and claim biblical authority for them when they happen to overlap with the Torah. The history of this process has yet to be written, and no one today, I think, understands it very well. However, in the brief life of our own country, we have seen more than enough of its effects. The early European settlers in this continent could scarcely make up their minds with regard to the Native American peoples, whether they were prospective converts to be saved, bodies to be enslaved, or Canaanites to be exterminated so that we could seize our "promised land." Even when the settlers opted for the first, they almost always demanded that Native Americans become culturally white in some significant way in order to enjoy God's gift of grace. The same ugly story can be told with regard to black slaves. The scenario is still being played out wherever the Church looks askance at some group of people because of their race or ethnic identity or sex or, I believe, sexual orientation.

We say to others, "You can be saved—if you will be like us." That is what Jewish Christians of the first century said to European Gentiles in the first century. Once the Europeans got in, they in turn did what they could to bar the door against others. Happily, God is ultimately unhindered by all this. God gives gifts as God pleases, and perhaps those who are unclean are readier to receive them. The danger, so far as salvation is concerned, is less to them than to ourselves. I do not suggest that God withdraws his grace because of our pride; but I think we, like the prodigal's brother, may become less and less able to rejoice in that grace and to enjoy the giver of it precisely because we are so much committed to admiring ourselves instead.

The Church, of course, has been encouraged in this sin by the world in general. The early Christians were in a great hurry to become respectable, and we cannot blame them when we understand that they lived under the threat of persecution; the appearance of respectability was not only their best defense but practically their only one. In the fourth century we became very respectable indeed, courtesy of the imperial family; and ever since then in the Western world, we have been not merely respectable ourselves but pillars of respectability. We take this so much for granted that we quite forget the incarnate God whom we worship was anything but such a pillar.

The Church has become the guardian of public morals. Quite possibly there was no helping that; but we still dare not ignore the perils implicit in this role. Our social analogues who guarded public morals in the first century were not Jesus or the Twelve but the Pharisees, the Sanhedrin, the priests, the elders, and the scribes. They were upholding the existing order, the order defined by the purity code. They were the insiders who said to the outsiders, "Unclean." Perhaps, in our own time, we cannot avoid this role altogether. But at least we should be aware of the temptation and be aware that our faith is being tested at its deepest roots. Whom do we want to keep out? And why do we want to keep them out? Who, here and now, is the prodigal? And what does the prodigal's brother want?

I said that AIDS has been problematic for the churches at least partly because early on AIDS was associated with people who have long been named unclean by the majority of American Christians. I mentioned IV drug abusers and gay men. I must add to the list Haitians and Africans, for we have not yet fully repented and been delivered from our long history of racism. I and other white Christians often see our sisters and brothers of color as less worthy or important than we. Even if we would be profoundly embarrassed to acknowledge such a thing in ourselves, this is apparent in the lukewarmness of our response. The result has been to label AIDS as a disease of the unclean and also, therefore, as an unclean disease.

That AIDS is now in itself unclean is evident from the panicky responses of people who are convinced, despite the utter absence of evidence, that they may catch the disease from casual contact. Children with the disease have been driven out of schools or cruelly isolated within them. Sick persons have been brutally deprived of housing or livelihood. The same reaction against what is defined as unclean that once permitted people to throw stones at lepers and force them to live on the margins of cities and villages now permits people to abuse those who have this new disease—or are thought to have contracted it or even thought to belong to one of the groups more likely than the average to do so. Nothing could possibly make the ultimate destructiveness of the division between clean and unclean more apparent.

How, then, shall the Church respond to the AIDS crisis, given that we are who we are? We are as divided as the Church of the first century and, at the most profound level, by the same issue. We who have been saved by grace would like to earn that salvation *ex post facto* by our works. Being religious people, we set up purity codes that say, "Being good means being like us." To call on the Church to give up such sins once and for all would be easy, but such an appeal would not be conclusive now any more than in the beginning. Truth to tell, the Church's ambiguities stem from substantive disagreements over precisely these issues.

Paul's solution to the first-century problems may be useful to us now. Paul found churches riven between those who flouted purity rules, whom he called "the strong," and those who insisted that everyone must keep them, whom he called "the weak." Paul agreed with the strong in principle. He did not believe that keeping purity rules could enhance one's salvation. How can anyone be more saved than saved? How can God love us more than he already has in giving the Son for us on the cross? On the other hand, Paul did not believe that flouting purity rules could enhance one's salvation either. To turn indifference to purity into a kind of good work is possible, too. Either course of action, then, was alright precisely as long as one did not pretend to earn what God had already given as pure gift.

Paul vehemently opposed in each group the desire to impose

its way on the other, for such impositions are meant to honor ourselves rather than God. To the strong at Rome he wrote, "Do not despise the weak"; to the weak, "Do not judge the strong." No one is to be deprived of his or her own sense of clean and unclean; but, what is much more important, no one is to impose that sense on anyone else (Romans 14). This would mean, in our case, that even Christians who regard AIDS sufferers as unclean are not free to withdraw from them and become uncharitable. That would be judging others. Even if we think of others as unclean, we, like Jesus, will minister to them, serve them, and love them. We will do so, not in an effort to make them like us, but with the intention of rejoicing in God's love for them, in God's reception of them as returning children, in God's running out to meet them as a loving parent.

A telling detail of Jesus' ministry is that he not only ate with tax collectors and sinners but he ate with them repeatedly. He was invited back. There for all of us, weak and strong alike, is the model for our ministry. We ought so to minister among all people that we will be invited back, particularly so that we can be invited back by the unclean, by the outsiders, by those most prepared to rejoice in the free gifts of God. This is not only for their sake but for our own. In so ministering to those we may see as unclean, we are rejoicing over God's free gift to them of love and care. As we learn to rejoice in what God has given them, perhaps we will even come to recognize and believe that God has forgiven us as well. Perhaps when we believe that God has forgiven us, we shall also dare to recognize and confess that our sins have been forgiven. And perhaps when we have thus repented of our sins we shall be ready to give up the wounded stance of the prodigal's elder brother and join the feasting and celebration. In the last analysis, ministering to people with AIDS may prove to be for our own benefit far more than for theirs.

Biographical Note

Louis Countryman is professor of New Testament at Church Divinity School of the Pacific (CDSP) in Berkeley, California. He holds three academic degrees from the University of Chicago and a theological degree from the General Theological Seminary in New York. In addition, he has done postgraduate study at Hebrew Union College. He was engaged in the parish ministry in Oklahoma and Ohio prior to his academic career, which has included appointments to the faculties of Southwestern Missouri State University and Texas Christian University, where he was associate professor of New Testament at Brite Divinity School before joining the faculty of CDSP.

He is the author of a scholarly study, *The Rich Christian in the Church of the Early Empire: Contradictions and Accomodations*. His book *Biblical Authority or Biblical Tyranny?* is written for clergy and laypersons wrestling with the issue of biblical authority in the contemporary church. Fortress Press published his book *The Mystical Way in the Fourth Gospel* in 1987. His most recent work, *Dirt, Greed, and Sex,* is a study of New Testament sexual ethics published in November 1988. Dr. Countryman is a member of the Lutheran-Episcopal Dialogue, Series III, and of the General Board of Examining Chaplains of the Episcopal Church.

Lifted to Holiness

Frederick Houk Borsch

William Countryman's essay offers a number of fine insights and a helpful framework with which to reflect upon the ambivalences many Christians feel in our understanding of the Church and its mission of outreach to others. In an earlier day, the question was put simplistically in these terms: Is the Church first and foremost an ark for the saved or a hospital for sinners? At least a part of every Christian probably wants a faith that demands something—a challenge to become a more caring human being, able to reach out beyond self-centeredness. Likely, we want the same thing for our Christian communities. We want more than a gospel of cheap grace that leaves us only where we are. Yet most Christians also know that the good news demands that we reach out to others with an extraordinary graciousness and compassion, that we recognize that all are sinners and all are justified by grace. As Presiding Bishop Edmond Lee Browning said (in what has proved to be the most controversial phrase of his tenure so far), there are to be "no outcasts" in the Church.

The parable of the weeds and wheat (Matt. 13:24–30) tells us something of the struggle in the very early Church, and quite possibly in Jesus' time as well, between those who wanted the community to be different than the sinful world and those who called for acceptance and inclusiveness.[1] Countryman rightly points to the parable of the prodigal son (Luke 15:11–32) as a way in which Jesus confronted those who were prone to make diligence and goodness into a barrier against accepting others. The parables of the one lost sheep and the ninety-nine (Luke 15:3–7; Matt. 18:12–14), the laborers in the vineyard (Matt. 20:1–16), and other stories of Jesus also illustrate his desire to encourage and cajole his contemporaries into a new understanding of the extraordinary graciousness of the invitation to God's Kingdom. I think E.P. Sanders is right to argue that Jesus was seeking to restore fullness to the community of God's people in preparation for the inbreaking of the Kingdom and the dawning of the new age.[2] What was startling about the manner in which

Jesus issued the invitation, both in word and action, was that he did not first demand a changed way of life but evidently expected that acceptance into the community would mean a new life. The story of Zacchaeus (Luke 19:1–10) becomes an enacted parable in this regard. That which most sets the new way apart is inclusiveness!

Countryman uses the story of the Pharisee and the tax collector to point up the reversal that can take place in the new situation. One may guess that in Jesus' own telling of this story the focus fell more sharply on the Pharisee. Hearers of the parable today are prone to see the Pharisee as a stock figure. He is the self-righteous prig, while the humble tax collector is the good guy. But most tax collectors of the time would have been seen as extortioners allied with the occupying Romans, while Pharisees were devout individuals who lived sacrificially and charitably. They were known for humility. These were the best people. One notes that this Pharisee even gives thanks to God that he does not live sinfully.

What then is wrong with the Pharisee? He apparently wants to establish his goodness and moral superiority over against others like the tax collector. By his aloof posture and condemning words he distances good people like himself from those who are seen to be in the wrong. In so doing he indulges a kind of self-fulfilling prophecy. Because the tax collector is a "bad" person, he cannot participate fully in the worship and community life of God's people, and because he does not participate in worship and community life, he is, therefore, a bad person. Jürgen Moltmann sizes it up in this way: the Pharisee "opens up a devilish gulf between himself and the tax collector, when he seizes the good for himself and pushes the other man into evil."[3] The shock of the parable is that the goodness of the Pharisee, which causes him to try to set the tax collector outside of the community, in Jesus' view makes the good man in fact the outsider to the true community of Israel. In this way the first make themselves last. "The tax collectors and harlots go into the Kingdom of God before you" (Matt. 21:31).

One ought not underestimate Jesus' anger over the attitude of the moral captains of society. Many Christians do not want to see Jesus as someone who became angry. Scholars tend to relegate some of Jesus' shrillness in the Gospels to a later stage of controversy between the new Christians and Jewish leaders. Nevertheless that Jesus had a core of passionate displeasure with those who use their moral power to try to make others outsiders is hard to gainsay. In telling a story like this, Jesus can be heard "taking sides with human beings in a concrete situation where the existing politico-religious structure has dehumanized people."[4]

Many of the Gospels' healing stories also can be seen as part of Jesus' concern to restore the wholeness of the community in preparation for the new age. Illness and physical disabilities often were considered a sign of God's displeasure, probably the result of sin. Jesus' healings are acts of power in the new age, signaling God's readiness to include seeming outcasts in the invitation to the new reign of righteousness.[5]

Yet once this invitation is accepted, a new way of life seems to be called for. No one earns the invitation, but acceptance is meant to change lives. Those who, like Zacchaeus, Mary Magdalene, Bartimaeus, and others, may have considered themselves unacceptable and unloveable now find themselves accepted, included, loveable and therefore at least beginning to be loveable—able to reach out in love to others. This is the power of the gospel. "Half of my goods I will give to the poor," Zacchaeus says, "and, if I have defrauded anyone of anything, I restore fourfold" (Luke 19:8).

While this transformation should be seen in the doing of God's will and not just in pious words (Matt. 7:21), the new teaching of Jesus lays special stress on changed attitudes. With respect to sexual ethics this is heard in the startling words, "I say to you that everyone who looks at a woman lustfully has already committed adultery with her in his heart" (Matt. 5:28). On first hearing, the saying seems almost absurd. Who can avoid natural sexual desires inbred by eons of evolution? The words are probably not directed toward impulse and desire but what one does with them. Lust intends to use the other person rather than respect and love him or her. Sexuality, surely we know, can be very selfish and destructive. It requires grace to make it loving. Followers of Jesus may be no more than beginners in the life of the new age; however, they are called to begin. This chiefly involves reaching out to others in loving and accepting ways; that attitude itself requires discipline and growth in the ways of a more unselfish, *agape* love.

Countryman is certainly right to point out that much biblical teaching that deals with sexuality cannot be directly translated into our societies because it presupposes attitudes different than ours regarding purity, the status of women, and a kind of ownership of others. Still, an underlying concern with a purity that calls for acceptance, vulnerability, and care for others is translatable, and this is what is meant to change in how disciples live their sexual lives as well as in other ways.

I have a hunch, however, that it is not the Bible that is causing so much difficulty in the acceptance and love of those whose sexual behavior is considered by some to be not proper or normative. The greater problem, I believe, lies in the area of natural theology and may affect the attitudes of those who do not consider themselves religious just as much as attitudes of those who do. This area is more difficult to deal with because it is not very well examined and often involves unspoken understandings. Persons who do not read the Bible literally may attempt certain literal readings from the natural world regarding divine purposes and law.

Genital sexuality, on such a reading, was made for one purpose: procreation. Sexuality used apart from that purpose is not just sinful; it is in some fundamental way wrong, by being out of keeping with the way things are and are meant to be. This reading of natural law causes official Roman Catholic theology to see as wrong any act of genital sexuality that by its physical character or use of so-called artificial means of birth control precludes at least the possibility of procreation. While this position is sometimes criticized for concentrating on the physical aspects of sexuality, more sophisticated presentations actually stress the aesthetic/moral dimensions. The use of genital sexuality apart from its created purpose goes against what is beautiful and good.

The power and appeal of this reading reaches far beyond Catholicism and Christianity. Although a number of people are willing to modify it by allowing contraception and giving the expression of mutual love an equal place as a purpose of sex, they would still insist that the only proper uses of genital sexual acts are in circumstances directly related to procreation, that is, between a married woman and man.

In conversations on this subject I often hear a deep-seated fear. If one can question whether this is the way things are and whether this is how God has made divine purpose known, then one admits the possibility that God's purpose may not be clearly knowable and even that there may be no order to Creation and no Creator. The concern, therefore, reaches far beyond even the powerful preoccupation with sexual conduct to the most fundamental questions about life.

Within the scope of this chapter, even to begin an approach to this fundamental concern of natural theology is difficult. One does recognize that sexuality seems to have retained a special status with respect to natural theology when increasingly one perceives that to read God's certain purposes in a world that includes disease, floods, earthquakes and malformed babies is at best difficult. One may notice, too, that those who might be considered highly permissive in their views of sexual behavior have their own curious natural theology. From their perspective, all that "comes naturally" is regarded as at least not immoral. Humans are fully part of the natural order, and what is done instinctively out of natural desire, they would claim, can be said to be good, especially if others evidently are not harmed.

Both of these natural theologies might be criticized allowing little room for the truly human. In a sense, both ask that human beings follow a pattern laid down for them in nature. Reason, planning, creativity, and sacrificial loving do not seem to have the highest roles to play. The role of grace in helping human beings transcend some of the brutish aspects of nature seems limited.

A better theology of sexuality for our time might well be less literalistic and more humble about our ability to read God's will and purposes from what happens in nature. The Creation may be an arena of considerable struggle and imperfection. Several branches of science are today discovering the complex interrelationship between chance and certain basic principles of existence. In some ways, nature begins to look both simpler and more complex than we ever imagined.[6] To some, this new view of things may threaten their ideas about God. But in interesting ways, a world of both chance and laws leaves place for creativity and responsibility that neither a deterministic world nor a random world would do.

Such a world may have fewer single patterns that all are meant to follow as the only way. But there can be considerable room for grace, and for reason and love guided by grace, to be ingenious in working to make life more humane and loving. In that context, more open to exploration and adventure, Christians may continue to sense, from out of the heart of life, a call to holiness in our sexuality as in all aspects of living. Through our sexuality we may not only participate in the creation of new lives but we may also learn about giving and receiving, caring commitment, faithfulness, vulnerability, sacrifice, and compassion—in other words, we may learn about genuine love.

Such love doesn't just happen naturally, although nature plays an important part. In the name of compassion and inclusiveness, the Christian faith does no one a favor by suggesting that almost anything goes and that all "life-styles" are just different. On the other hand, there may be little or nothing that *agape* love cannot lift to holiness.

References

1. On the interpretation of this and several of the parables that follow, see F.H. Borsch, *Many Things in Parables: Extravagant Stories of New Community* (Philadelphia: Fortress Press, 1988).
2. See E.P. Sanders, *Jesus and Judaism* (Philadelphia: Fortress Press, 1985).
3. Jürgen Moltmann, *The Power of the Powerless: The Word of Liberation for Today,* trans. M. Kohl (San Francisco: Harper & Row, 1983), p. 96.
4. Jon Sobrino, *Christology at the Crossroads: A Latin American Approach,* trans. J. Drury (Maryknoll, N.Y.: Orbis Books, 1978), p. 92.
5. See F.H. Borsch, *Power in Weakness: New Hearing for Gospel Stories of Healing and Discipleship* (Philadelphia: Fortress Press, 1983).
6. See, for example, James Gleick, *Chaos: The Making of a New Science* (New York: Random House, 1987).

Biographical Note

Frederick Borsch earned baccalaureate degrees at Princeton and Oxford, where he also earned a master's degree. His degree in theology is from the General Theological Seminary. He went on to take a doctorate at the University of Birmingham in England. He embarked upon an academic career after serving a parish in Oak Park, Illinois. He tutored at the Queens Theological Seminary and was a lecturer at the University of Birmingham. In this country he has served on the faculties of Seabury-Western

Theological Seminary, the General Seminary, and was dean, president, and professor of New Testament at the Church Divinity School of the Pacific. He was Dean of the Chapels at Princeton University at the time he was elected Bishop of Los Angeles, a post he assumed in June 1988.

The Realm of the Pure and the Impure

Patricia Wilson-Kastner

In clear, calm language Professor Countryman has outlined his diagnosis of the common human tendency that underlies the churches' inconsistant response to those afflicted with AIDS. Church people have, as Countryman reminds us, befriended the sick and, at the same time, called AIDS "a divine judgment on people whom the church has rejected."

The conflict emerges from that fundamental tendency in humanity to separate and distinguish "us" from "them," the pure from the impure. Jesus identified the major and central problem with purity rules: they lead the "pure to glorify themselves" even as the impure know that they must "seek and glorify God." Unhappily, purity legislation returns inevitably to infect the Church. The AIDS crisis has enabled the Church to apply clearly its rule of separating the pure from the impure by objective behavior, homosexual relationship. Thus AIDS is a sign and manifestation of unclean behavior, a clear mark of impurity.

I would add to Countryman's analysis that the stigma of unclean behavior is applicable to the other groups in the United States that are major sufferers from AIDS: IV drug users, the women who are their partners, and the children who come from their unions. Intravenous drug users are, in the eyes of many, the willing participants in what is often termed a "plague"; despite legal changes, deep in our culture lies a sexism that regards women as inferior and unclean. Furthermore, children with AIDS, although usually portrayed sympathetically, share in the generally inferior status of children in our society and are connected by birth and blood with the avowedly unclean.

If one adds to this mix the reality that the new growing population of people with AIDS are poor, and frequently either Hispanic or black, new factors of uncleanness and exclusion complicate the situation. Sexual behavior, race, economic status are all elements that add to the separation and impurity of people with AIDS in the minds of many in the Church. As this is written, the scene is shifting. The constant factor is that almost all people with AIDS come from sectors of society already regarded by the majority as inferior and set apart by their behavior or their very being to some degree. AIDS functions as an objective sign that manifests the truth to everyone: these people are unclean. I think Countryman's analysis of the conflict between the clean and the unclean has implications far beyond the division between gay and straight.

Professor Countryman suggests that because the Church will not, in fact, give up its purity rules, Christians will continue to regard people of homosexual orientation as unclean. Therefore he programmatically proposes a solution that follows the approach Paul lays down in his letter to the Romans. "Do not impose your strength on the weak," the apostle suggests to the condemning heterosexual. Imposing one's way on the other is self-glorification rather than worship of God. Instead, even if "we think of others as unclean, we, like Jesus, will minister to them, serve them, and love them." If we follow this way, Countryman offers the hope that we will come more fully to believe not only that God has forgiven them, the impure, but that God also loves and forgives the pure, who also have much that God forgives them.

Refusing to Live in the Realm of Grace

When I first read Countryman's essay I was moved and full of admiration. I still feel touched by his suggestions and deeply affected by his solution to a painful and divisive problem within the Church. However, besides praising him, I would like to raise a basic question about his approach. Putting my objection in simple terms, I think that Countryman offers us a practical, ad hoc solution to a theological and religious problem.

Ought the Church to be in the business of setting up purity laws and deciding who's in and who's out on the basis of such laws? Who determines what the laws of behavior are, and who makes the decision about who is and is not clean and unclean? Countryman does not address these questions in any substantial way. Rather, he appears to accept as a given the human tendency in the Church to divide the pure from the impure. As a practical suggestion he advises people not to impose their particular vision of strength and weakness on the other. Let those who consider themselves strong minister to the weak.

Countryman supposes that such ministry of the self-identified strong and pure to the weak and impure will change those who minister into more compassionate persons, more aware, he implies, of their own weakness and dependence on God's grace and forgiveness. I suspect that Countryman's practical and pastoral approach would indeed be helpful and constructive for those who would honestly and humbly join in such ministry. Even the most rabid homophobic soul or despiser of IV drug users would be transformed by a loving encounter with the one he or she had condemned.

Countryman's solution has pragmatic Christian wisdom to recommend it, not to mention apostolic authority. But even in the face of such formidable recommendations, I would insist that one can read the situation another way and offer a theological-religious response to the theological-religious challenge of those who judge people with AIDS to be unclean and impure. I would like to explore an alternative.

I begin my argument by asserting that I think William Countryman is a kind and gentle person, much nicer than I am going to be. My approach tackles the division of the Church into clean and unclean, pure and impure. I agree that the Church tends to behave that way and that the AIDS crisis has allowed Christians so inclined to do much condemning of those they consider impure and unclean. Just because people tend to make such judgments, however, does not mean that we as Christians ought to condone their action.

I think Countryman's assessment of Jesus' refusal to be bound by the purity laws of the Torah and the Pharisaic tradition is correct. Their approach does tend to lead to self-glorification. Even more fundamentally, a religion based on purity inevitably becomes anthropocentric. Our energy is absorbed by *our* observance of the law and *our* purity. We are centered on ourselves, not on our relation to God. (I want to leave aside the question of the historical adequacy of the Gospel portrayal of Pharisaism within Judaism. The Gospel certainly identifies a temptation within Judaism and Christianity to assume that our behavior justifies us before God.)

None of us wants to live in God's realm of grace—not at first, at least. Humanity's primitive religion is very much like our earlier human relationships: "O God, give me what I want, when I want it." As we mature enough to realize that we do not get everything we want, our religion grows to the next stage: "O God, give me what I want because I do what you tell me to; I am good." Our focus is still on ourselves and what we want; our behavior is self-justification for deserving good from God. Our religion is anthropocentric (selfish, to be more blunt), and God's role is to be our parental rewarder.

Whatever else Jesus proclaimed, at its core was a religious approach centered in a relationship to God that was initiated by God's absolutely free and unconditional love. Christianity has struggled long, hard, and sometimes unsuccessfully with its Founder's insistence on the primacy of God's love, which reaches out to us to evoke a response of love and dedication to God. Today's AIDS crisis provides people with one more excuse to judge others on the basis of behavior, to use language about the pure and the impure, to divide the world into the good and the bad, into the righteous whom God rewards and the sinners whom God hates and punishes.

Countryman is too kind when he permits people to cling to a perception of God as rewarder of our good. Just because the Church has allowed new purity rules to be set up around issues of sexuality and drug use does not mean that we can allow such beliefs to continue unchallenged. Please note that I do not say any sexual behavior is fine or that IV drug use is good. My point is merely that we cannot begin any helpful reflections with a God whose relationship to us consists of rewarding the good and punishing those who behave badly. If we do not begin with God's grace and mercy, we are not yet Christian.

An Alternate Vision

As Countryman suggests, today we Christians are in urgent need of a religious approach to the AIDS crisis that will enable us to feel and to act with compassion and with active and positive concern for all persons with AIDS. Whereas he proposes a Pauline-based practical approach that will lead us to new religious-theological perspectives, I would like to try to press us to a more direct theological position, which also owes something to Paul and perhaps even to Jesus.

We need to begin with grace, not sin or good deeds or even our willingness to suspend judgment. When I speak of grace I do not mean primarily God's forgiveness of us or favor toward us but rather the Spirit of God dwelling in us (Rom. 8:9–17). This Holy

Spirit unites us as one in the Church and gives us each a variety of gifts (Eph. 4:1–16). For our purposes the essential element of the Spirit of God's activity among us is the Spirit dwelling in us. That is, grace is a relationship. Grace is not primarily a transaction in which God passes judgment on us but rather a name given for the mystery of God's coming to dwell with each of us who are God's children.

In the Catechism of the *Book of Common Prayer,* in the section on baptism, we read, "The inward and spiritual grace in Baptism is union with Christ in his death and resurrection, birth into God's family the Church, forgiveness of sins, and new life in the Holy Spirit."[1] Grace is a relationship between God and the believer, a relationship in which God's own life becomes the center and core of the believer's life. This grace is the source and power of our capacity to pray, to respond to God and to others, to do what good we can, and to hope for eternal life. Only in this grace of God dwelling in us is our peace and righteousness.

Laws and distinctions based on purity and impurity are based on objective observation of actions. But the ethics of the gospel emerge from the relationship of the human being to God and to others (e.g., Mark 7:14–23). For the Christian, our participation in the risen life of Jesus is founded on and rooted in the new relationship God establishes with and in us through the indwelling of the Holy Spirit, not in certain behaviors or deeds.

The AIDS crisis is a genuine crisis of faith for many people because it calls them to judge and be judged. They are called to extend love, compassion, and service to people who are often marginalized in society—gays, IV drug users and their sexual partners, children of the poor. How to draw the lines? Consider this example: Let us suppose that all children are innocent by definition. As a consequence one would think that they would automatically be the objects of compassion. Yet more lines of judgment are drawn in community discussions: What is the danger of infection to me? We see people immediately operating with two principles of judgment at work: (1) Are the victims good enough for me to approve of, and (2) do they pose no real danger to me?

By making such judgments the community finds itself judged. Instead of beginning with our common relationship in God and asking how we can best act out that relationship, people have begun with fearful self-concern and self-righteousness and made protection of themselves the primary motivation of their actions. All of us can sympathize with fear and the urge for self-protection, and we would defend people's right to reasonable prudence and health precautions with each other. But the underlying issue, about wise, careful, and caring love, is obscured by our human exclusiveness and refusal to accept our mutual relationship rooted and grounded in the presence of God in us.

As Christians we want all of our behavior, our words, deeds, thoughts, feelings, to emerge from the grace and presence of God in us, not from fear and self-centeredness. I suggest that this starting place points out to us certain values to guide our lives rather than a list of laws that encourage us to include or exclude ourselves or others.

If grace is the most basic reality of our lives, we are called to live as people in communion with God and with each other. If we are truly living in the presence of God, with God's life intertwined with our own, how shall we live out our natural needs and desires? our sexuality? our eating and drinking? our ambition? our desire for comfort and companionship? Rather than predetermining certain kinds of behavior as automatically good or evil (either from natural law theology or from lists in the Bible we think we understand), would we not be better off seeking guidance from God, as made known to us in the Word and in our world? How do our lives reflect faithful love, redemptive judgment, peace, unending joy, and perfect communion?

Rather than divide or allow others to divide the world into clean and unclean, we Christians can provide the world a great gift by showing others how we live in grace and love. We do not ask if the other is clean or unclean, weak or strong. We receive with joy the news of God's redeeming love to all of us and the presence of God in us. Our response to one another is based not on how the other behaves or has behaved or even what is the safety or risk factor to me. Our response springs from our awareness of the Spirit of God in us binding us all as one. We are grateful for God's grace and love to us and know that any judgment to be made is God's work, not ours. (We are humbly aware that from God's perspective we may be the object of judgment, rather than the one doing the judging.)

Our task, as Christians, is to live out the grace we have received, to express with joy and enthusiasm the gift of God we have received. In many ways this call is much harder than the ethical response Countryman suggests. But I would like to propose that the Church reflect seriously on its need to manifest to the world its thanksgiving for the grace we have all received, rather than to spend its time asking, "Mirror, mirror, on the wall, who is the worthiest one of all?"

According to the Scriptures, God alone is holy (Rev. 15:4). We share in God's holiness, not by doing certain things that are pure or impure, but by receiving into our lives the Spirit of God who comes to us. This grace of our relationship to God is the source of our community with one another in simplicity and compassion, not in judgment and self-righteousness. In its response to the AIDS crisis, may the Church choose such a grateful response to God in its care for all of God's children, for we are all children of the same divine grace.

Reference

1. *The Book of Common Prayer* (New York: Church Hymnal Corporation, 1979), p. 858.

Biographical Note

Patricia Wilson-Kastner is Trinity Church Professor of Preaching at the General Theological Seminary. She is priest associate at Christ and St. Stephen's Episcopal Church in Manhattan and author of a number of books and articles. She earned her baccalaureate and master's degrees at the University of Dallas and her doctorate from the University of Iowa.

Part 3.
Thinking about Sexual Ethics

Introduction: Thinking about Sexual Ethics

In the minds of many people in our society, the adjective *religious* is a code word for someone who doesn't think sex is very nice. Each semester, during the nearly two decades I have taught human sexuality on secular college campuses, I have avoided "coming out of the closet" as a clergyman until I had gained credibility as one who had something useful to say about sexuality. Upon discovering my priestly vocation, my students acknowledge they would not have registered for my course had they been aware I was a clergyman.

Most secular people believe the institutional church has little of constructive value to say about sexuality or sexual behavior. The actions of some officials of the Christian churches have forfeited credibility on this subject, particularly in the past two centuries (see William Countryman's comment regarding Christian dialogue with Jews and the gay community, in Part 2). In the eyes of secular Americans, the rigid and erroneous stance of the Roman Catholic hierarchy on the subjects of contraception, abortion, and the use of condoms continues to disqualify institutional Christianity from speaking on sexuality. Lest this statement be viewed as harsh, I hasten to add that my comments refer to the institutional hierarchy; I do not refer to the responses of many Roman Catholic clergy and religious who have established hospices for persons with AIDS and sero-positive infants, demonstrating unconditional love and compassion in the AIDS crisis.

This loss of credibility is tragic because Christians have good news to proclaim on the subject of sexuality! This loss is particularly tragic in light of the splendid work by Christian scholars as seen in the books listed in the annotated bibliography. Little funding has been available since the midseventies for scientific research in human sexuality, but an important corpus of scholarly philosophical and theological work has been produced, much of it by Christian thinkers.

This work has been done in the "ivory towers" of the seminaries but awaits dissemination to the proverbial "people in the pews" of local churches. The AIDS epidemic offers rich opportunities for this to be done. We Christians and Jews believe that sexuality is God's gracious gift to humanity. We must proclaim the good news that the love of God can be mediated in the sexual loving of human beings. In our sexual intimacy we experience a unique transcendence. The people of God must not forfeit our right and our opportunity to be special advocates of this gift of God the Creator.

Norms of Faithfulness

In the extemporaneous discussion at the conference, Ann Lammers comments on the penultimate paragraph of her presentation in which she speaks of applying the norm of covenant fidelity. She raises the question, "How could we treat this norm in such a way that it wouldn't be a weapon to exclude or punish people in the actual circumstances in which they find themselves?" She speaks of her own relatively dehumanizing marriage followed by several years as a single person, and her progressive struggle to understand commitment. Based on psychological theory and her own experience, she offers a model of normativity that is directional rather than absolute. She draws from an image fashioned by Teilhard de Chardin describing a deep-sea diver rising toward the surface who with each stroke draws closer to the light.[1] Each moment the diver is closer to the light than the moment before. "That doesn't mean that the person who is even closer to the light has the right to say to you, 'The place where you are now is bad.' Or that you have the right to say to someone else who is struggling up, 'The place where you are now is bad, I reject it.' Look instead at the direction in which the swimmer is moving." It would be wrong to move toward a deeper darkness, a less faithful life.

"I couldn't in my own life situation go back now and reenter a patriarchal marriage. I couldn't resume a frenetic life as a single person. That doesn't mean I've finished learning about fidelity. Maybe someday I'll say I couldn't return to the way I lived in 1988. One has to look at the direction of one's own swimming."

Lammers urges us to avoid saying, "Nothing but covenant marriage or a total lifetime commitment will do, and we condemn you for your present partial commitments. We also can't say, 'I can't possibly talk to you until you change your sexual orientation because you are beyond the pale.'" But she continues, "It's not true that we have no insight as a Christian body about what God would wish us to be in our sexual lives. If we say we have no norms at all, we are abandoning people who come seeking guidance. Neither response is a way of joining people to Christ." She urges that norms of faithfulness be applied to the longitudinal direction of people's lives.

The Peril of Seeing God in the Norms

Fred Borsch describes the possible causes of the fear of some who are solely reliant on a certain kind of natural theology for their sexual norms. "One of the reasons why homosexuality and some other forms of sexual behavior which are 'outside the norm' are so threatening to a number of people who are reading this natural theology is because their natural theology is crucial to their understanding of God's existence. It isn't just that they are homophobic; they may be or they may not be; but I don't think we always understand them correctly if we just see them as wrong or misguided. They are saying '. . . if this isn't the way it is, then there is no God and Creator,' and that is, of course, very threatening. Not only are they losing God but they are losing their sense of order. Unless we find some way to address that concern, or that issue, which again is much more difficult to address because it is often unspoken, I think we are not going to connect with the concerns of some of those people. [They are crying out] 'THAT IS NOT THE WAY IT IS!' . . . When we try to suggest by a different kind of perspective—by grace, by gospel perspective, by entering into other people's lives—one can see different possibilities of love and sexuality and so forth that need not be so threatening to God's existence but [could] help us to a deeper understanding of God."

Sexuality and Spirituality

Oliver Vannorsdall proposes a central question for twentieth-century society on the subject of sexuality: "How do we incarnate our sexuality into our spiritual life?"

For Christians, the starting place for the answer to this question is found in our perceptions of God. We base our sexual ethics on our understanding of the sexuality of God. Does one perceive God as sexual? erotic? heterosexual or homosexual? punitive or nurturing? Yahweh God the Creator was understood by the ancient Jews as not being sexual at all. Yahweh God did not utilize sexuality to create but created by *logos,* by word and will. Our human sexuality is not an aspect of God, but it is a creature of God, a divine gift given to humanity as the radical solution to the problem of loneliness (see Genesis 2).

What do we believe about the sexuality of God? Lammers finds the answer to that question in the Old Testament book *The Song of Songs.* Vannorsdall comments, "God's eros yearns for us, yearns for relationship, and the emphasis in Philippians [is on] the God who empties him/herself as spirit and is desirous of impregnating us [answering the question of the sexuality of God]. The source of our desire for relationship is the result of Spirit. God is erotic and loves beauty and loves pleasure." Vannorsdall refers to Alice Walker's novel in which Shug believes that God gets annoyed when we don't appreciate the color purple.[2]

We are cocreators with God, not only in reproducing the species (note that "procreation" means participating with God in creating) but also in the process of fulfilling our potential by becoming the person God created each of us to be. William Miles, an HIV pastoral researcher in the infectious disease clinic at Fitzsimmons Army Medical Center, describes how he urges each patient to accept his own identity—a real challenge in the military environment that "forbids" military personnel to be gay. "I have found that the ministry that is the most valuable, that I have been led into, is to help our patients become who they are sexually, to at least be able to admit it to a small group of us, to be and become who they are. At that point we can help them have an attitude of wholeness and wellness in the face of this virus that we fight."

Lammers affirms this process of self-acceptance and identifies it as the starting point in a much larger process. The individual makes a major step toward wholeness by accepting his or her own identity and sexual orientation; the next step for many people is to reveal one's self to one's family. The challenge in this process of self-acceptance is for the family to identify itself to the world as one that includes a gay person. They have to decide if they are willing to say who they are, truthfully, to their intimates. A similar and perhaps parallel process takes place with the acceptance of the fact of HIV infection. Lammers describes the process as "individuation, truthtelling, which spreads, from that one moment; it has a reverberating, widening effect. And the more we can allow, tolerate, truthfulness without fearing that we are going to be annihilated, the healthier we are spiritually."

Rosa Escobar: Thank you for this opportunity to talk a little bit about sexuality and us: Hispanic and black. We believe that sexuality is something we must hide; it is something even though, if you like I will do, is ugly. We don't tell it to anyone. As a parent, when we raise our children we told our children to hide sexuality, the same way we were raised, not to let anyone know what was going on. When it is coming to the point that one of our children became ill with AIDS, we are so scared! But so scared that our neighbors, our family, our people surrounding us know that we have a gay person in our family, or we have a drug addiction child in our family that we hide that even more. When that person starts to get sick, we try all kind of remedies, everything we can before taking that person to the hospital, because taking that person to the hospital it means that everybody going to know what is going on in our family, and we don't want that to happen. So I believe that from the black and Hispanic perspective the situation is even worse because of the difficulties to have people around us to help. We don't even go to our priest telling our priest what happen in our family, we are so scared that you won't believe it.

The Bronx and Harlem are one of the places that have most AIDS population. The situation of sexuality and how we hide that sexuality from our children, that is our culture. We are very hard to broken down. We need the help of everyone, of all ethnic groups.

Risking Conversion

Gene Robinson, a priest of the diocese of New Hampshire, speaks of his fear of being overwhelmed by the possibility of an "anything goes" ethic of sexual behavior. He describes how his own personal growth usually came when he was willing "to jump from a safe shore into a raging river, with the hope that I can make it to the other side. . . . It also conjures up for me the image of the slaves being led out of Egypt by Moses." He wants to know how Moses persuaded them to take that risk. But despite

Moses' persuasive powers, many of the slaves wished to return to oppression in Egypt. After a period of wandering, they found being dependent upon God terrifying. Robinson asks Lammers, "How do we get people to jump off the safe shore into these raging waters? What do we need for protection? You pointed to autonomy and fidelity as possible standards; you said we need a ruled Christian ethics, a new agreement about moral norms. I take that to mean you believe there is some safety in the raging waters, but how do we get people to jump in, and what are those 'ruled places' that make it a protective environment?"

"There are always two moments in talking about conversion. [The first is] the jumping into the raging waters—giving up one's idolatrous certainties, one's habituations," Lammers responds. "You can't hold onto rules as you are jumping into the raging torrent, but you must jump, and you hold onto the relationship to Christ, however that transcendance is interpreted at the moment. It might simply be an awareness that in the deepest darkness, God is. There is that moment of dissolution of rules. . . . We in the Church are always between the necessity of being reconverted, [between] judgment and conversion, when the rule structure becomes a self-created God-substitute. Worship Christianity? Worship the Church? No, no. We need to repent of that, jump into the torrent of uncertainty.

"And then there is another moment that says, 'From the certainty of the relationship to Christ, and from the fact that jumping into the torrent didn't end life but gave a new life, one comes out on the other shore.' Then you have the adjudication of daily relationships, and the coherence of the community that can say, 'These are the scriptures we read in church.' . . .

"We don't say that absolutely any act or behavior is acceptable, because some of them hurt. Even if we don't know it at the time, we know from later experience that it hurts. Adultery is a good example. It hurts. The secrecy, the lying, the split loyalty, the keeping one's self in the dark, . . . there are these ambiguities in the adulturous relationship that we don't have to find out from scratch every time. There are some things we know ahead of time; there are some rules that apply, a theoretical lens that can be used; these things are likely to crop up. . . . Because we know them, because human beings enact the same kinds of drama and don't make it up from scratch, it is possible to make generalizations and even governing rules. The real problem is how we then teach what the rules are.

"We can connect them up with peoples' own inner experience and say, 'Here's why it matters: not because Daddy or Mommy or the Church says so, but it matters intrinsically.' Sin actually hurts people; that's why there is a rule against it."

The metaphor of leaping off into the raging waters is used repeatedly during the discussion. Vannorsdall points out that "change seems to take place when we are on the edge, or forced on it, as with AIDS. It is forcing all of us to relook at our sexuality and what we mean by that and where we want to go with it. I don't know how many times I have heard persons with AIDS say, 'This has been the most meaningful time of my life.' There is growth, and unfortunately it comes with slaps in the face."

Armando Rios: When you are dealing with AIDS in the Latin community you find yourself not only giving an AIDS 101 course but also a health care course. Unless they are third or fourth generation Latin Americans, they know very little about their bodies. Girls are not taught about their menstrual cycles. When they refer to their bodies when they go to the doctor they say, "I'm having problems down there."

Being gay, like in any culture, is very much a taboo in the Latin community. But if you're a "flaming queen" you are much more readily accepted by your family and the rest of your community than if you do not look gay. [Effeminate gay men are less of a threat to other men than a masculine gay man.] Even before we talk about sexuality we have to talk about the taboos, and it's difficult.

Irwin Rubiola: I agree with what you say, but also one of the things we have to remember is that in Latin America and the Caribbean, the predominant religion was Roman Catholic. Many of those myths come through the church. The Episcopal Church must look into that before it starts breaking those taboos. Recently, while studying religion and sexuality in the Latin community, I asked, "How often do you talk about religion at home?" It was almost twenty-four hours a day. "How often do you talk about sex at home?" It was discussed at home only when a newborn was arriving: "It's a male; it's a female—and you don't need to know any more about it."

Harmless, Yet Wily

Throughout the discussion, concern was expressed at how much easier it would be to deal with AIDS if we could skirt the issue of homosexuality. National Episcopal AIDS Coalition president Thad Bennett's concern was more pervasive: He is concerned that the Church skirts the issue of sexuality itself. He is concerned that, picking up the metaphor of jumping from the bank into the raging river, the Church will urge people to stay on the bank and not risk growth. "We have to talk about jumping into the water: we have to talk about gay sexuality, sexuality in the black and Latino community that is different from talking about sexuality in the Anglo community—and how as a Church do we talk about that stuff? How do we find a way within Christianity to talk about safer sex practices, the diversity of the sexual experience? Can we empower the Church to recognize that the Church is the one place in our society where people can trust? that when there is a conversation about jumping into the water, about sexuality, it's going to happen in an appropriate way? The Church is the place where you are guaranteed you won't drown; there is going to be our faith, the love of God, that will prevent us from drowning!"

With a cautionary tone, Lammers reminds us Jesus could not talk to some towns. She urges that we stop identifying the Church with the institution. "Let's not be limited like that. The Holy Spirit has tricks up her sleeve. God is absolutely full of tricky ways of getting the truth told. If we don't, the stones will. It's not just a matter of how to get the institutional church to shape up and tell the truth, how to get every parish in this national Episcopal Communion to become a safe place: that would be wonderful! Every parish and every family *should* become a safe place to be who you are and say it out loud and describe what you have actually done and been through and what it has cost you and what you have gotten from it: it's devoutly to be wished."

However, she continues, "Knowing that every parish is *not* a safe place, be very careful where you spill your guts. Don't assume; don't project. Just because the man/woman is a rector and has a collar on, don't assume that person is a safe person to talk to. Hear that person's story. Is he/she telling the truth about self? Find out whether true stories are being told, and if it is a place where true stories are being told, it is probably a safe place to start telling your own. Is this the time, the place? We can get terribly hurt in the family. It is good to be childlike but don't be infantile in your projections onto the church that it must instantly become the perfect family. It's not going to; it's just too human for that.''

References

1. P. Teilhard de Chardin, *The Divine Milieu: An Essay on the Interior Life* (New York: Harper & Row, 1965).
2. A. Walker, *The Color Purple* (New York: Washington Square Press, 1982).

New Dimensions in Human Sexuality

Robert T. Francoeur

Any discussion of AIDS today inevitably forces us to wrestle with issues of sexuality, although that subject is peripheral to the syndrome itself. This accident of circumstance diverts attention from the central issue of the virus, to the peripheral issues of the sub-groups of society here in the United States who have contracted the virus, and happen to be gay or bisexual. So, with this assertion that AIDS and its consequent diseases are not "gay diseases," I plunge ahead into the topic of sexuality.

The attention directed to homosexual orientation as a result of the AIDS epidemic illuminates the fact that six to twelve million American men and three to seven million American women are exclusively or predominantly homosexual in their orientation and life-style. Many people have been diagnosed with HIV who were thought to be heterosexual, but close examination of their histories reveals that perhaps fifty million men are more or less bisexual in their sexual relations.[1] We cannot deal effectively with AIDS policies, education, and ministry unless we also face the reality of life-styles, orientations, and behaviors that many, perhaps most, Americans might prefer to ignore and leave hidden in the shadows of denial and silence. To avoid the issue of sexual orientations is to avoid reality.

As Christians, we are forced to reexamine our religious traditions and our moral principles. Unless we want to claim that every question about human sexuality has been specifically addressed and answered by divine revelation in the Bible, we are forced to reexamine our Christian heritage once again. Paul, Augustine, Aquinas, Luther, Calvin, the early councils, Vatican I and Vatican II, and the Lambeth Conferences suggest we don't have all the answers; let me propose an outline for reexamining the Christian meaning of Creation and sexuality.

Five hundred years ago, in an essay entitled "On the Dignity of Man," Renaissance writer Giovanni Pico della Mirandola described God telling man about the meaning of our Creation:

> We have given to you, Adam, no fixed position, no form of your very own, and no gift uniquely yours, so that you may feel as your own, have as your own, and possess as your own seat, the form and gifts which you yourself shall desire. Other creatures have a limited nature. They are confined within laws written down by Us. In keeping with the free will and judgment We have given you, you are not confined by any bounds. You will fix the limits of nature for yourself. We have placed you at the center of the world, so that you may more conveniently look around and see everything in the world. You are the molder and maker of yourself. Restrained by no narrow bonds, according to your own free will . . . you shall sculpt your nature in whatever shape you prefer. . . .[2]

The Genesis myth speaks to the core reality of our being human. Genesis does not refer to an event in some distant once-upon-a-time. Could God who is and who is without distinction of past, present, and future, "have done" or "said" anything except in a human interpretation that must talk about past, present, and future? A divine Eternal Now can only "be saying" or "doing." The Creation accounts speak of an irresistible, irreversible stream of becoming in which each of us is mutually, intimately, and inescapably involved together in the ongoing creation of cosmogenesis. "We are at once the creators of our reality and the victims of our creation."[3]

Defining or Describing Our Sexuality

Many Christians today still speak from a fixed Aristotelian philosophy of nature. In this unbiblical, pre-Galilean, pre-Darwinian, pre-Einsteinian worldview, the Creator created from above and outside. These Christians see themselves as custodians of divine Creation, as curators awaiting the return of the Infinite Museum Owner. (Remember the story of the careful servant who dug a hole and hid the master's money, told in Matthew 25?) Other Christians struggle to be good and faithful servants willing to risk in order to realize more fully their vocation and to define the reality of their own potential. They take their inspiration from the Spirit and Word that move through matter. They are the co-creators who through faith, human experience, and risk strive to listen and respond to the challenges of a world and humanity moving toward the unfolding of the ultimate Kingdom. While the curators make rules for behavior in the museum, the co-creators strive to bring forth the living art works that will decorate the Kingdom.

The Judaeo-Christian tradition is a tradition precisely because, in every historical and social circumstance, the thinking faithful have brought to bear the best interpretation of the current realities in correlation with their interpretation of tradition as they have inherited it. Thus, truth in the Judaeo-Christian tradition is a dynamic process to be discerned and formulated rather than a static structure to be received.

The Bible is misunderstood and misused when approached as a book of moral prescriptions directly applicable to all moral dilemmas. Rather, the Bible is the record of the response to the word of God addressed to Israel and to the Church throughout centuries of changing social, historical, and cultural conditions. The Faithful responded within the realities of their particular situation, guided by the direction of previous revelation, but not captive to it.[4]

To define is to limit, to control. Those who try to define life, human nature, human sexuality, and the human experience attempt to control or hold power over life, nature, and experience. Those who would define life imply that they control the Kingdom and access to it. This approach challenges the fullness of the mystery of the Incarnation. It rejects the Word who is becoming flesh in our sexual nature. Are we willing to imprison both humanity and the Epiphany of the New Adam/Eve in a narrow museum constructed out of our patriarchal cultural biases and our lack of human imagination, faith, and courage? Are we so concerned about maintaining our power?

Because we are the pivotal, controlling element in the development of the Whole Christ, because we are immersed in this ongoing cosmic process, we cannot stand outside that life to examine, define it, and judge it. At most we can only make statements about some part of it based on our observations and experiences. Our participation colors everything we report. "Reality, inasmuch as it has any meaning at all, is not the property of the external world [existing] on its own, but rather it is intimately bound up with our perception of the world—our presence as conscious observers."[5]

The only way to cope with this partiality of vision and experience is to share with others the multitude of our partial experiences. Life can only be comprehended through shared, trusting, and truthful consciousness. The experiences each of us has in our sexuality and our relationships are as valuable and as valid as those of any other human because they are our experiences. To ignore or eliminate the data and experience of any person or group of persons because they do not fit our preconceptions and definitions prevents us from more fully participating in life. Since life is a single developmental process from beginning to *pleroma,* approaching life through shared consciousness requires that we include all the components of the human experience, the scientific, historical, religious, political, aesthetic, and cultural experiences of individuals and groups, past and present.

Our prevailing traditional definitions of sex and sexual relations belong to an outdated worldview, or at least to a *weltanschauung* that is fast retreating before the evolutionary perspective of contemporary knowledge. Sex and sexuality no longer define property rights, either the property rights of males over females and children or the legitimate passage of property through male heirs. Children are no longer central to the power of either the individual parent or the state. As patriarchy and the sexuality it defined fade, new forms of sexuality and human sexual relations gradually emerge.

Our challenge is to make these new forms and relations more humane and more responsible than our traditional sexuality was. This means combining the best of traditional values—kindness, cooperation, equality, justice for all levels of society—with the metamorphosis of a more personalized and egalitarian society. This means replacing the submission of Eve to Adam; the marital primacy of Eden; the dualism of Paul, Augustine, and the early fathers that exalted celibacy and barely tolerated marital sex; and the traditional inflexibility of sex roles and life-styles with a much less genital, more sensual and pluralistic understanding of sexuality and nurturance.

From Creation and Sex as Work to Creation and Sex as Play

Whether it was impregnating, making babies, or, more recently, mutual, multiple orgasms, the productive "goal" of our sexual work ethic has prevailed in our patriarchal view of sexuality. Human sexuality was at first tolerated and slowly embraced within marriage because it allowed us to produce new members for the Kingdom. Theologically, and as a culture, we are still uncomfortable celebrating the pleasure of sexual relations. Only recently have theologians like Sam Keen suggested that we replace the work ethic of sex with an aesthetics of playful sexuality as a more human and appropriate value system.[6] Alex Comfort maintains that sexual play is "the healthiest and most important human sport."[7] In *The Joy of Sex,* Comfort added that "sex is the most important form of adult play. . . . The rules are only those of childplay."[8]

Play is creative. Alex Comfort once mentioned to me an Indian myth of Creation not as work but as the gods engaged in a playful game. Heraclitus said, "The course of the world is a child at play, moving figures on a board, back and forth; it is the kingdom of a child."[9] In keeping with this paradigm, William Phipps suggests that "playing requires that we take the world, life and creation neither more seriously nor more lightly than it demands."[9a]

Children learn by playing; why can't adults also learn by playing? Play and games suspend the reality we think is out there. They give us a critically new perspective, a new insight into interpersonal frontiers. In *Total Sex,* Herbert and Roberta Otto describe sexual play as "spontaneous, free-flowing, creative, joyous, or pleasure activity. Relatively devoid of structure and without the element of competition, sexual play is essentially a leisure activity with directions emerging from within the person."[10] In *The Feast of Fools,* Harvey Cox urged a festive affirmation of living as an alternative to the daily routine of work, convention, anomie, and mediocrity.[11]

Physicist Brian Swimme argues that "the difference between humans and other primates [lies] in the ability of the human to make play its dominant activity throughout a lifetime. . . . To say that play is essential to the human species is to corroborate what creative scientists, artists, and great saints have understood as central to their own activities. Play, fantasy, the imagination, and free explorations of possibilities: these are the central powers of the human person."[12] What lies behind play, fantasy, imagination, and free exploration of possibilities but the ecstasy and epiphany of the Transcendent Other?

A New Dimension

In the West, since the beginning of recorded history, males have defined the nature and the meaning of human sexuality. Centuries separated the rare female voice, from Sappho to Eleanor of Aquitaine's courtly love, and the mystic orgasms of Theresa of Avila. In the late 1800s, women began to speak out more forcefully on the meaning of their sexuality, on marriage, and on the rights of women. When she dared to question the patriarchal definitions, Victoria Woodhull, an advocate of social freedom for women, free love, divorce, and decriminalized prostitution, was immediately labeled "Mrs. Satan." Harriet Beecher Stowe, Emma Goldman, "Red Kate" O'Hare, Edith Wharton, Elizabeth Stanton, and Margaret Sanger were dismissed as dangerous anarchists or socialists.[13] In the 1960s, the voices of women finally forced a hearing when *The Feminine Mystique* awoke a movement we now take for granted.

The advent of effective, simple oral contraceptives undoubtedly helped society listen to what women had to say about sexuality because it allowed women to experience sex without risking pregnancy. Years before the pill, Max Marcuse had warned that the separation of human sexual relations from procreation would pose a major threat "to authoritarian life and culture."[14] Our contraceptive technologies challenge the traditional patriarchal images of human sexuality, both religious and secular, by demolishing the procreative work ethic of sex. They open the door to an aesthetics of human sexuality in which sensual play transcends the marital dyad to eroticize friendships of many different types. Thus did women's liberation, feminism, the sexual revolution, and gay liberation open a new era. No longer could the churches and our theology of sex ignore the voices of sexual minorities and woman.

In describing the feminization of sex, Barbara Ehrenreich, Elizabeth Hess, and Gloria Jacobs confess,

> First, we challenged the old definition of sex as a physical act. Sex, or "normal sex," as defined by the medical experts and accepted by mainstream middle class culture, was a two-act drama of foreplay and intercourse which culminated in male orgasm and at least a display of female appreciation. We rejected this version of sex as narrow,

male-centered, unsatisfying. In its single-mindedness and phallocentrism, this form of sex . . . cannot help but remind us of the dangers and ambiguities of heterosexuality. At best, it reminds us simply of work: "sex" as narrowly and traditionally defined is obsessive, repetitive, and symbolically (if not actually) tied to the work of reproduction.

We insisted on a broader, more playful notion of sex, more compatible with women's broader erotic possibilities, more respectful of women's needs.[15]

The implications of "women's broader erotic possibilities" are important because they open up new dimensions in our understanding and experience of human sexuality. The real difference between the male and female experience of sexuality is much deeper than the genital differences. The work of James W. Prescott, a neuropsychologist, indicates that women have a finer and more extensive integrating neural network in the cerebellum of the brain than do men. Prescott traces this richer development phylogenetically to the stimuli of extensive nurturing and body contact females have experienced for countless generations back through our primate ancestors in infant care and child rearing.[16]

In a similar vein, biobehavioral scientists talk about a difference in prenatal programming of the neural tendencies in men for a lower threshold of sexual response to visual stimuli while women have a higher visual threshold and respond more quickly than men to touch. It is not the genital superiority of women that is important so much as their more humane and broader experience of sexuality in terms of touching, playful sensuality, nurturance, and communion.[17]

The Values of a Sexuality Reexamined

Opening to new dimensions our understanding of something as fundamentally human as our sexuality forces us to reexamine traditional values in order to identify the underlying perennial principles that were incarnated in the sexual values of the past and that we now must distill and reincarnate in a new value system.

Incarnating human sexuality in an aesthetic paradigm is an open attack not just on patriarchal values but also on the power structure those values have supported. It is thus an attack on both consumeristic capitalism and authoritarian governments, both civil and religious.[18] Comfort agrees with Herbert Marcuse that "the acceptance of sensuality and the widening of its focus to include not one but many others" will likely be correlated with a new sense of social justice, nonpossessiveness, nonexploitation, ecological concerns, and the eroticization of friendship.[19] A shift in sexual values brings with it an across-the-board shift in all our values and attitudes because of the very intimate and personal nature of sexual values. This is a vital but too often ignored point. Christian ethics should be a seamless garment, to borrow a phrase from Cardinal Bernardin of Chicago. Our sexual ethics share the same foundation as our whole moral outlook on life. Too often sexual ethics have been seen as the touchstone of Christian morality.

Let me begin a brief exploration of how we might articulate the perennial human values in our sexuality of the 1990s by tapping three prophetic, but generally ignored, efforts of recent years.

In 1970, the United Presbyterian Church in the U.S.A. issued a work-study document, "Sexuality and the Human Community."

> We regard as contrary to the covenant [of Jesus] all those actions which destroy community and cause persons to lose hope, to erode their practical confidence in the providence of God, and to lose respect for their own integrity as persons. Clearly, such actions are not susceptible of being cataloged.

> By the same token, those sexual expressions which build up communion between persons, establish a hopeful outlook on the future, minister in a healing way to the fears, hurts and anxieties of persons and confirm to them the fact that they are truly loved, are actions which can confirm the covenant Jesus announced.[20]

To be human in this Christian perspective, sexual expressions and relations should enhance rather than limit the spiritual freedom of the individuals involved. They should be vehicles for expressing that love commended in the New Testament—a compassionate and consistent concern for the well-being of the other. They should expand the creative potential of persons and be the occasion of joy. They should open to persons that flow of grace that will enable them to bear their burdens without despair.

In 1977, the American Catholic Theological Society of the United States issued the results of a commission study of the "serious discrepancy" between the static, patriarchal sexual values consistently articulated by the Vatican and the more person-oriented sexual values of American Catholic theologians and laity. Though it was officially condemned by the Vatican, it is apparent from a variety of sociological surveys and polls that the majority of American Catholics accept as valid the eight basic values outlined in that study and reject the Vatican's positions on contraception, premarital sex, and divorce.

In this Roman Catholic statement eight values are highlighted. All human relations, especially those that involve sexual intimacy, should be self-liberating and other-enriching—not just nonexploitive but actively concerned with the needs of the other. They should strive to be honest, faithful to whatever commitment is made, responsible, life-serving, and joyful. Above all, sexual relations should be transcendent, leading individuals beyond themselves to communion with others, the world, and God.[21]

Shortly after the American Catholic Theological Society report was published, one of its coauthors, Anthony Kosnick, joined me on a panel with the Reverend Anne Ross Steward, a Methodist minister; and Lester Kirkendall, author of a "New Bill of Sexual Rights and Responsibilities" issued by the American Humanist Association.[22] After three hours we were surprised at the depth of our agreement about what the human meaning of human sexuality should and could be if we were willing to set aside our traditional biases and preconceived definitions and faced the challenge of reexamining our human sexuality.[23]

Ten years later I find similar perennial values in what I believe is the equally prophetic "Report on Changing Patterns of Sexuality and Family Life" from the Episcopal Diocese of Newark, New Jersey.

Some Key Issues

Relationship/recreational—nonprocreative—sex includes a wide variety of experiences, including masturbation, contraceptive marital coitus, oral stimulation, anal penetration, and homosexual, bisexual, and lesbian relationships. (The penetration of the anus, practiced in both heterosexual and homosexual relationships, although by a minority of both groups, has become identified as the practice most likely to result in the transmission of the AIDS virus. The risk is only slightly reduced with condoms, as they were not designed to withstand insertion into the anal sphincter.) The challenge for Christian ethicists, theologians, church leaders, and the faithful is to reincarnate the essence and values of the Christian vision in these experiences, which are an undeniable part of human life today.

Masturbation. For young children, adolescents, single persons of all ages, married persons, gay men, and lesbians, masturbation can be a recreating of one's energies; a playful release of tension; a mutual pleasuring shared with a partner; or an exploration of one's own sexuality. In traditional terms, "wasting the seed" was condemned as immature, hedonistic, narcissistic, and egotistic.

In the patriarchal work ethic, masturbation is totally immoral, a disordered act, an unnatural enjoyment of sexual pleasure that God reluctantly uses to induce adults to assume the burdens of parenthood. Masturbation was believed to drain the body of its vital fluids and weaken it so that we cannot work.[24] In defending his "Teenage Chastity Bill" a few years ago, Senator Jeremiah Denton (R-Alabama) said masturbation and premarital sex are "imprudent self-indulgence" that may be "one of the greatest threats to the survival of our nation" and its moral fabric.[25]

In 1984, the 30th General Council of the United Church of Canada took a prophetic stand on the Christian value of masturbation, admitting, "We cannot assume that our teenagers are paralyzed from the neck down. Nor can we tell them 'no genital sex before marriage' unless we have some good reasons to give them. . . . Parents particularly need to be aware that masturbation for the teenager may be a healthy sexual outlet." Masturbation is a playful way to explore our bodies and their sensual/ sexual potential built into them by the Creator God. We need to know how to pleasure and nurture our own bodies before we can relate sexually with another person.

Homosexualities. Some Christians define and condemn homosexual relations as immoral and disordered. This ignores the preponderance of evidence indicating that homosexual, heterosexual, and bisexual orientations are due to two factors, factors described by the noted researcher John Money as "love's maps", which determine sexual proclivities throughout the individual's life: (1) biochemical, neural, and hormonal templates laid down in the fetal brain, before birth, and (2) the individual's often subconscious and chance response to an unpredictable and unique combination of triggering experiences and stimuli encountered in childhood and finalized during puberty in love maps that are very resistant to change.

Several prophetic responses to the new understanding of sexual orientations have emerged from a vocal gay community and the research of sexologists. In asking about the morality of homosexual and lesbian relationships, the Catholic Theological Society report concluded "it bears repeating, without provision, that where there is sincere affection, responsibility, and the germ of authentic human relationships—in other words, where there is love—God is surely present."[26] Joan Timmerman, professor of theology at the College of St. Catherine in Minnesota, suggests that "the same criteria should be used to judge homosexual relationships that are used in evaluating non-marital heterosexual relationships. The morality that governs friendships, alliances, and relationships between persons of any sort is applicable to sexual non-marital relationships."[27] Timmerman, I should mention, cautiously opens the door to pre-, post- and nonmarital coital and noncoital relations, so her statement cited here is more open to homosexual relations than it might seem if isolated from its context.

In discussing the morality of homosexual relations, the Newark Episcopal report reaches a similar conclusion:

> From the perspective of Jesus' teaching regarding the Realm of God, all heterosexual and homosexual relationships are subject to the same criteria of ethical assessment—the degree to which persons and relationships reflect mutuality, love and justice. . . . The commitment to mutuality, love and justice which marks our ideal picture of heterosexual unions is also the ideal for homosexual unions. Those who would say homosexuality by its very nature precludes such commitment must face the fact that such unions do in fact occur, have occurred and will continue to occur. The Church must decide how to respond to such unions.[28]

The challenge for the churches and theologians is to listen and understand before trying to respond to the realities of homosexual and lesbian couples and their needs. The report continues:

> Changing patterns of sexuality and family life confront pastors and congregations with new challenges and opportunities for understanding and for ministry. Rather

than arguing about these issues we need first to listen to
the experience of those who are most directly involved.
Where homosexuality is concerned, fear, rejection, and
avoidance by the heterosexual community is common and
entrenched. We believe that pastors and congregations
must meet members of the homosexual community person to person. The first step toward understanding and
ministry is listening. We need as much as is possible to
bracket our judgements and listen to persons as they are.
The Church needs to acknowledge that its historical tendency to view homosexual persons as homosexual rather
than as persons has intensified the suffering of this 5%–
10% of our population.

Listening opens the door of hospitality, which has so
long been firmly shut. Such words as ministry and hospitality, however, still suggest a relationship of inequality,
we and they. As such they perpetuate the image of the
Church as separate from the homosexual community. In
fact, however, we believe that the Church should be as
inclusive of homosexual persons as it is of heterosexual
persons. In this light, all the normal avenues of inclusion
should be available to homosexual persons. . . . Ideally,
homosexual couples would find within the community of
the congregation the same recognition and affirmation
which nurtures and sustains heterosexual couples in their
relationships, including, where appropriate, liturgies
which recognize and bless such relationships.[29]

Other sexual expressions. Our traditional sexual value system has led us to deny the sexuality and sexual needs of other
minorities besides homosexual and bisexual persons. We have
also tried to ignore and deny the sexuality of children, adolescents, the disabled, those in prisons, and older persons, especially those in nursing homes, residential institutions for the
aged, and hospices.

We know next to nothing about the normal, healthy, psycho-
sexual development of children. In other cultures, sexual re-
hearsal play is openly accepted. That is not the case in Western
civilization, where we have adopted a punitive response to any
sexual expression during childhood and adolescence. This may
have been functional in ages past when children, apprenticed
out at age seven, were considered to be young adults and when

marriage occurred in the early teen years. Today, with sexual maturation occurring in the early teens and marriage increasingly postponed until the early or midtwenties, we need to reexamine our Christian response to the sexuality of children and adolescents. Timmerman asserts that "in a society in which experiential knowledge of sexuality is lacking in any ritual form, it is understandable that young people will seek such knowledge through experimentation with each other."[30]

How should we respond to this reality? Some have suggested that we create religious rituals and rites of passage to recognize sexual maturation and to acknowledge and support the commitments of sexually active single persons. Some have also urged that we examine the apparent connection between antisocial and paraphilic sexual expressions in adults and the attempts by society and parents to repress and punish the gradual emergence of sexual expression in young persons. Adult paraphilic behavior can often be traced to early repressions that traumatize and divert a child from developing a normal lovemap.[31]

We also know very little about couples who are struggling with commitment, fidelity, and Christian values in nonmarital unions, in sexually open marriages, in comarital relationships, and in intimate networks. Man-sharing in the black community and extended families headed by single women supported by female relatives are a reality the Church quietly ignores. It is apparent that the monolith of monogamous marriage supplemented by single spinsters, common only a century ago, has evolved into a pluralism of adult life-styles and relationships. How do we respond to this reality?

New dimensions in commitment and fidelity. The traditional, lifelong, sexually exclusive monogamy based on premarital virginity and the bonding of several children now constitute a small minority among American adult life-styles. Well over half of our adult population between ages eighteen and thirty-five are single persons, most of them sexually active. One in two marriages ends in divorce. Reconstituted or blended families outnumber traditional monogamous families. For example, 48 percent of all school children in the state of Texas are part of single-parent families. The proportion of cohabiting couples continues to increase. In this context, interpersonal commitment and fidelity in a relationship may no longer be defined in terms of sexual exclusivity but rather as something much deeper and more valuable. Commitment and fidelity appear, in fact, to be taking on new dimensions even as we agonize over the changing texture of family life. More inclusive definitions of commitment and fidelity appear to be emerging, in terms of mutual responsibilities to the ongoing growth of multiple relationships as more and more men and women experience serial, and sometimes simultaneous, multiple relationships.[32] The AIDS epidemic has apparently reduced the number of multiple relationships in the gay community, but it is not clear to observers of American society that relationship practices have changed significantly among the heterosexual population.

For the most part these developments are taking place while religious institutions deny and ignore the changes, thus forfeiting the opportunities to provide guidance and shape the emerging value systems. There are exceptions, however.

In August 1988, the United Church of Canada approved the ordination of homosexuals and others who have sexual relations outside marriage. While the focus is on the homosexual issue, the resolution also gave church approval to intimate relationships between men and women outside of marriage so long as they are based on a "commitment" by those involved.[33] This, I believe, represents an open-ended, prophetic description of Christian commitment and covenanting in today's world.

A story in the *National Catholic Reporter,* describing the recent Lambeth Conference of the bishops of the Anglican Communion, states that in 1866 Bishop Massaia of Ethiopia asked the Vatican's Holy Office whether a Roman Catholic priest could accept polygamous families into the church and whether slave traders could be given the sacraments. In a classic closed definition, the Vatican replied that "polygamy is prohibited by divine law but slavery can be allowed under natural law."

The decision of the 1988 Lambeth Conference to reverse its hundred-year-old resolution forbidding the baptism of polygamists and their families represents a prophetic response to our ongoing development as sexual persons. As Bishop Njugana of Kenya said during the debate, "Christ did not come to break families but to strengthen them." Traditionalists urge continued condemnation of polygamy, sexually open marriages, and gay unions. But they will tolerate divorce and remarriage, which some aptly call "Christian serial polygamy."

The Reverend Gene Hillman, a Holy Ghost priest working in

Africa, has urged the Vatican to adopt the Lambeth position because it respects the openness of Christ. Until the "perfect" model for marriage is found, what else can we do except struggle to incarnate basic Christian principles of love, commitment, concern, joy, honesty, trust, fidelity, and transcendence in relationships that vary from culture to culture, from society to society, from age to age. Is there only one acceptable model, or can humans follow different paths to intimacy, love, and transcendence?[34]

A New Sexual Perspective

The philosophical/theological question we need to ask is whether we want to remain trapped in the Platonic/Aristotelian worldview of cyclic time and eternal archetypes, what Mircea Eliade called "the myth of the eternal return,"[35] or whether we are willing to take seriously the linear time of the biblical vision with the very nature and essence of things being created by us as we move toward the fullness of time.

Excluding self-destructive or exploitative behaviors or relations, no single path, life-style, or way of relating is in itself better or less meaningful than any other. The totality of human sexuality can only be expressed partially and in different ways by each of us at different times in our lives. Each of us takes his or her own unique path in responding to the erotic potential of the whole universe and everything in it. William Stayton speaks of this interaction as a "panerotic potential" in which we can find nurturance and sensual whole-person communion in many different outlets: in the sensuality of our own bodies, in the world of nature, with other persons of both genders, and in the mystical, the cosmic, and the spirituality of a transcendent deity."[36]

In a time when the human race faces the threat of a nuclear winter, the greenhouse consequences of our industrial imperative, starvation, poverty, and economic exploitation, to assert pleasure—especially sexual pleasure—as a legitimate social goal is risky indeed. But the "real issues" just cited only reflect our vast, collective separation from the body, from the earth, and from other life on it. This dichotomy within the human spirit has made it impossible for us to delight in ourselves and each other. We live in a condition of estrangement, from our own true nature, and from each other; an estrangement that contributes to alienation from God. If we want to solve the "real problems," are we not then obliged to rethink pleasure as a human goal and reclaim it as a human project?[37]

Intimate human relations have their roots and spirit in the synergistic, multifaceted, pluralistic, sensual, and erotic interactions of persons with other persons and with everything they encounter within the cosmic womb. Only by embracing the full sensuality of the human potential can we assure our full development as humans. To be human we need to regain our cosmic roots and sensitivities, to embrace the sensuality of nature's womb, to celebrate the nurturance of all caressing touches of the hand, the hair, the wind, the water, the warmth of fire and sun, and the cool dew. We need to rejoice in the creativity of playful eroticism. We need to listen to diverse voices with a discerning spirit. Only then may we hope to experience communion in the spirit and the fullness of our God-endowed potential as sensual/sexual persons.

Five hundred years after the first Renaissance began, we are facing a new Renaissance. Once again Pico della Mirandola's challenge comes to the fore. Today, however, the challenge of sculpting human nature has been extended. Now it is not just Adam, Man, who is describing the fuller meaning of human sexuality. Today, Eve also accepts the challenge as women contribute their experiences. The married have been joined by the unmarried and postmarried. Heterosexuals have been joined by homosexuals and bisexuals, as persons of all sexual orientations contribute to our understanding of human sexuality.[38]

References

1. This estimate is based on current U.S. Census population figures and the standard interpretation of the Kinsey and more recent studies that indicate between 5 and 10 percent of males are exclusively or predominantly homosexual in their orientation while 3 to 6 percent of females are exclusively or predominantly lesbian in their orientation. Overall, Kinsey found that 46 percent of American males could be classified as more or less bisexual in their sexual experiences and fantasies. See A.P. Bell, M.S. Weinberg, and S.K. Hammersmith, *Sexual Preference: Its Development in Men and Women* (Bloomington: Indiana University Press, 1981), and A.P. Bell and M.S. Weinberg, *Homosexualities: A Study of*

Diversity among Men and Women (New York: Simon & Schuster, 1978).

2. P.D. Mirandola, *On the Dignity of Man, One Being, and the One, Heptaplus,* trans. C.G. Wallis, P.J.W. Miller, and D. Carmichael, modernized by R.T. Francoeur (1485; reprint, Indianapolis: Bobbs-Merrill Educational Publishing, 1965), pp. 4–5.

3. F.A. Wolf, *Taking the Quantum Leap* (San Francisco: Harper & Row, 1981), p. 142.

4. N.S.T. Thayer et al, *Report of the Task Force on Changing Patterns of Sexuality and Family Life* (Newark, N.J.: Episcopal Diocese of Newark, 1987), p. 9.

5. P. Davis, *Other Worlds* (New York: Simon & Schuster, 1980), p. 12.

6. S. Keen, *To a Dancing God* (New York: Citadel, 1970), p. 26.

7. A. Comfort, *Sex in Society* (New York: Citadel, 1966), p. 26.

8. A. Comfort, *The Joy of Sex* (New York: Crown, 1972), p. 85.

9. Fragment 52 (Diels). From Jürgen Moltmann, ed., *Theology of Play* (New York: Harper and Row, 1972), p. 15.

9a. W.E. Phipps, *Recovering Biblical Sensuousness* (Philadelphia: Westminster Press, 1975).

10. H.A. Otto, and R. Otto, *Total Sex* (New York: Peter H. Wyden, 1972), p. 299.

11. H. Cox, *The Feast of Fools: A Theological Essay on Festivity and Fantasy* (Cambridge: Harvard University Press, 1969).

12. "[A] species denied its true habitat perishes. . . . What is the true habitat of the human? Adventurous Play. A human denied this habitat of adventure and surprise is denied the opportunity to become truly human. . . . Adventure is an adventure into the unknown. True play is without predetermined direction or definition. We are to explore, to learn, as deeply as we can to probe and experiment, and above all to laugh. . . . Perhaps the entire natural world is a tremendous party, a festival, and we the long awaited champagne" (B. Swimme, *The Universe Is a Green Dragon* [Santa Fe: Bear Press, 1985], pp. 120–23).

13. B.I. Murstein, *Love, Sex, and Marriage Through the Ages* (New York: Springer Publishing, 1974), pp. 368–80.

14. M. Marcuse, *Die ehe; ihre physiologie, psychologie, hygiene*

96 Thinking about Sexual Ethics

und eugenik; ein biologisches ehebuch (Berlin & Kholn: Msarcus & Weber, c. 1927).

15. B. Ehrenreich, E. Hess, and G. Jacobs, *Re-making Love: The Feminization of Sex* (New York: Anchor Books/Doubleday, 1987), p. 183.
16. J.W. Prescott, "Body Pleasure and the Origins of Violence," *The Futurist* 9(1975):642–74. Also, "Developmental Origins of Violence: Psychobiological, Cross-Cultural and Religious Perspectives" (An invited address presented at the annual meeting of the American Psychiatric Association, May 4, 1983).
17. J. Money, *Gay, Straight, and In-Between: The Sexology of Erotic Orientation* (New York: Oxford University Press, 1988).
18. M. Kamenetzky, "The Economics of the Satisfaction of Needs," *Human Systems Management* 2(1981):101–11.
19. A. Comfort, "Sexuality in a Zero Growth Society," in R.T. and A.K. Francoeur, eds., *The Future of Sexual Relations* (Englewood Cliffs, N.J.: Prentice Hall, 1974), p. 57.
20. United Presbyterian Church in the U.S.A., *Sexuality and the Human Community* (Philadelphia: United Presbyterian Church, 1970), pp. 11–12.
21. Kosnick et al., *Human Sexuality: New Directions in American Catholic Thought* (New York: Paulist Press, 1977).
22. L.A. Kirkendall, "A New Bill of Sexual Rights and Responsibilities," *Humanist Magazine* 36(1976):4–6.
23. R.T. Francoeur, "A Positive Humanist Statement on Sexual Morality," *Free Inquiry* 7(Winter 1986–87):15–17.
24. J. Money, *The Destroying Angel: Sex, Fitness and Food in the Legacy of Degeneracy Theory, Graham Crackers, Kellogg's Corn Flakes and American Health History* (Buffalo: Prometheus Press, 1985).
25. W.E. Phipps, "Masturbation: Vice or Virtue?" *Journal of Religion and Health* 16(3)(1977):183–95.
26. Kosnick et al, *Human Sexuality,* p. 218.
27. J. Timmerman, *The Mardi Gras Syndrome: Rethinking Christian Sexuality* (New York: Crossroad, 1986), p. 107.
28. Thayer et al., *Report of the Task Force on Changing Patterns of Sexuality,* p. 10.
29. Ibid., p. 11.
30. Timmerman, *Mardi Gras Syndrome,* p. 106.

31. J. Money, *Lovemaps: Clinical Concepts of Sexual/Erotic Health and Pathology, Paraphilia, and Gender Transposition in Childhood, Adolescence, and Maturity* (New York: Irvington Publishers, 1986).

32. A.K. Francoeur and R.T. Francoeur, *Hot and Cool Sex: Cultures in Conflict* (New York: Harcourt Brace Jovanovich, 1974), pp. 118–31.

33. J.F. Burns, "Canadian Church Approves Homosexual Ministers," *New York Times,* August 28, 1988, p. 19.

34. P. Windsor, "Acceptance of Polygamists Called 'Right Step,'" *National Catholic Reporter,* August 26, 1988, p. 36.

35. M. Eliade, *Cosmos and History: The Myth of the Eternal Return* (New York: Harper & Row, 1959), pp. 88–91.

36. W.R. Stayton, "A Theory of Sexual Orientation: The Universe as a Turn On," *Topics in Clinical Nursing* 1(1980):1–7.

37. Erhenreich et al., *Re-making Love,* pp. 207–8.

38. James B. Nelson expanded on this point in relating incarnation and embodiment when he wrote that "the church must do its ongoing theological and ethical work with a high sense of responsibility. Fresh insights from gay Christians, from feminist theologians, and from those secular scholars who frequently manifest God's 'common grace' in the world remind us of the numerous ways our particular sexual conditionings have colored our perceptions of God's nature and presence among us. If the Protestant Principle warns us against absolutizing historically relative theological and ethical judgments, so also an openness to continuing revelation should convince us (as it did some of our ancestors-in-faith) that 'the Lord has yet more light and truth to break forth'" (J.B. Nelson, *Embodiment* [Minneapolis: Augsburg, 1978], p. 181).

Biographical Note

Robert T. Francoeur brings to this subject an expertise gained by study and experience in several fields. After earning a theology degree at St. Vincent's College in Latrobe, Pennsylvania, he was ordained a priest in the Roman Catholic Church and then taught high school biology, physics, and theology. Later he studied at Johns Hopkins and Fordham Universities, and earned his doctorate in experimental embryology at the University of Delaware. He is recognized as an expert on the evolutionary synthesis of Teilhard de Chardin and has served as president of the Chardin Society. He is a prolific author with a lengthy list of books on Chardin, evolution, biology, and human sexuality. His college textbook, *Becoming a Sexual Person,* is regarded by many as the best in the field. He has presented more than seventy papers at meetings of the Society for the Scientific Study of Sex; the American Association of Sex Educators, Counselors and Therapists; the World Future Society; the World Congress of Sociology; the American Association of Pastoral Counselors; the National Council on Family Relations; the World Congress of Sexology; and numerous other medical and religious groups. He presently holds the position of professor at Fairleigh Dickinson University.

Acknowledgment: The author is deeply indebted to the Reverend Joseph Casey, a friend and colleague at Fairleigh Dickinson University, who has served as a sounding board, critic, and collaborator in developing and refining many of the ideas in this paper.

Rules of Play in Sexual Ethics

Ann C. Lammers

Robert Francoeur makes several good points and makes them so well that I can only applaud them. These points include the potential for joy and playfulness in all of human experience, including sexual life; strong evidence that human sexual orientation is not chosen but determined before or soon after birth; and the fact that modern feminist theory has made contributions to a more humane view of sexuality. All these are vital and valid aspects of his essay, and I am grateful to him for arguing them so convincingly. It is especially important to remember that God's gifts are precious and embodied life a miracle to be celebrated, especially in the AIDS epidemic which confronts us so painfully with issues of death and loss.

I want, however, to focus on an aspect of Francoeur's contribution that may be in danger of unbalancing the rest. His theological anthropology is the part that poses the danger. Its almost unlimited enthusiasm about human creativity needs to be balanced, in my opinion, by a cautionary word about the realistic limits of human power and goodness. I am a bit worried, though, lest in urging a more modest anthropology on which to base a Christian ethics of sexuality, I may fall back into the rigid punitive ethics that both Francoeur and I are at pains to refute. Let me explain what I think are the dangers on either side.

Francoeur rightly rejects a theory of human life based on a Platonic and Aristotelian substantialism that many modern theologians have abandoned. This theory is still being put forward by official Catholic spokespersons, however, as a foundation for Christian sexual ethics. Recent statements from Rome on sexuality and reproduction all assume a teleology that says in principle what sex is "for" and then expounds moral rules consistent with those ends. The metaphysics of such a perspective comes from a certain kind of neo-Thomism frequently used by conservative Catholic writers as a barricade against change. It is a philosophy that allows medical and sociological findings, and self-knowledge based on experience, no real place in the debate.

Francoeur is right to criticize a sexual ethics grounded in rigid archaic anthropology and administered punitively to chilling effect. Christian sexual doctrine affects the spiritual lives of believers. Conservative ethics tends to straightjacket some in an orthopraxy based on abstractions and to humiliate others for being faithful both to their own sexual direction and to their sexual partners. Still others are threatened with the loss of sacramental fellowship.

A church that behaves this way is an oppressor, an institution of spiritual tyranny. It would be perverse *not* to criticize such a church, wherever it appears. The Roman Catholic Church, in the person of its local theologians and ethicists, does not really match such a portrait, of course, and least of all in this country. But the power of a strict hierarchical polity and the fact that the discipline of the Vatican Curia stretches overseas create situations of a sort that allow one to recognize the institution in the portrait. I am delighted that Francoeur approves of some of the work done at Lambeth, and I hope Anglicans and Roman Catholics will continue to collaborate at all levels of conversation. In responding to his argument I find we are standing, as it were, in neighboring counties on the same map.

The Episcopal Church at this point in its history seems committed to an open debate on sexual ethics. This commitment entails the public airing of moral tensions between and among Christians, even to the point of sometimes being embarrassed by what people put in print. In its moral diversity and messiness the Episcopal Church reflects contemporary society. Some would like the church to reject the diversity of moral opinions and establish a uniform position. But the existence of diversity does not mean the church has abandoned its mission or lost its soul, only that it cannot impose moral agreement from above.

By a slow, painful process of dialogue, debate, and mutual encounter, "the mind of the church" comes to light, not by the apparently more efficient—but easily abused—hierarchical imposition of uniformity. On the other hand, the word *pluralism,* which is often invoked in a favorable sense to describe both the Episcopal Church and society at large, is useful only as long as its sociological neutrality is recognized. Mere "pluralism" is not the gospel; it describes the current conditions in which the gospel must be preached. We must now suffer through disagreements about Christian sexual ethics, not for the sake of "pluralism" as such, but hoping that in time we will have a new agreement about moral norms, based on a better understanding of the gospel and of each other.

In the diversity of positions on sexual ethics in the Episcopal Church today, I notice at least two approaches, or methods, commonly in use. These include *legalism*—rational and scriptural—and *subjectivism*—theological and experiential. Each of these approaches has its dangers. When the legalists go wrong they behave like the bandit Procrustes, chopping up life to fit their prior conclusions. When the subjectivists go wrong they obscure the outlines of reality like a certain vine rampant in the south that muffles trees, fences, and telephone poles indistinguishably. Fearing legalism, Christian moralists sometimes propose subjectivism in its place. But we must be careful lest, fleeing the bandit, we succumb to the kudzu.

Rational legalism is based on principle, as we see in official writings of the Roman Catholic Church. This approach defines sexual morality *a priori*, based on an abstract teleology whose disembodied ahistorical qualities Francoeur rightly criticizes. Scriptural legalism in evangelical circles, on the other hand, locates biblical injunctions concerning sexual behavior and applies these commands more or less literally to the acts and relationships of present-day people. Either use of legalism tends to ignore individual experiences, the observations of pastors, doctors, and families, and recent findings of science that shed light on human capacities and behaviors.

One of the cures for legalism, as I mentioned, is subjectivism. Francoeur's argument, as I read it, rests on subjectivism of two kinds, which I am calling theological and experiential. Theological subjectivism forms his primary argument.[1] This position begins with the fact of Creation and says that human beings have been given the task of progressively cocreating ourselves and our world. The innate goodness and playfulness of human beings, especially in our sexual lives, is Francoeur's special application of the broader principle that we are cocreators with God.

A danger accompanies theological subjectivism, however. There is a tendency to overemphasize the glorious birthright of cocreativity, while failing to give equal time to the human plight of finitude and sin. In so energetically affirming human goodness, Francoeur appears to forget that we are not only gifted and powerful but also slaves of our habits and destroyers of what we ought to preserve. It would seem necessary for a Christian to confess that the shadow of sinfulness pervades all of life, including sexuality, and that its roots extend into the very freedom and creativity that make human life potentially so glorious.

One reason why this admission of personal sin is necessary is that if we deny the personal roots of sin we are tempted to project all evil without remainder onto social oppressors (e.g., by focusing on the violence of homophobia). Thus we pretend to settle the question of evil while maintaining our own goodness. A doctrine of individual righteousness invites us to play down our need for salvation and divides humanity into two classes: righteous sufferers (who would be creative if only they were not so wickedly oppressed) and wicked tyrants who oppress them. This projective pattern becomes problematic whenever we feel ourselves vulnerable and badly treated or identify ourselves with others who are victims. Then we tend to ascribe all innocence and pain to ourselves, all power and freedom to the enemy.

In his essay's unqualified claims about personal righteousness, I fear Francoeur may lead us astray, even if he does so with the best of motives. He emphasizes *homo ludens* and *homo faber*—humanity as the player and the maker. He admires the insights of Renaissance humanism, which appreciated the elegance and beauty of the human creature as if for the first time.[2] Because his is a creation-centered theology, Francoeur takes God's playfulness, creativity, and freedom as warrants for celebrating the same qualities in humanity made in the image of God. But a Christian must ask, If we are cocreators, are we coredeemers as well? If we are playful, creative, and free, will we be saved by our playfulness, creativity, and freedom?

This doctrine of self-redemption is never stated in Francoeur's essay, but it is implied by the sheer exuberance of his diction and it is nowhere denied. Sin is mentioned mainly under the rubric of social oppression and violence toward minorities and individuals. The essay hints at a doctrine of personal sin, sin rooted in personal freedom, only once. This hint intrudes as qualification to a declaration of moral tolerance that would otherwise be absurdly broad: "*Excluding self-destructive or exploitive behaviors or relations,* no single path, life-style, or way of relating is in itself better or less meaningful than any other."[3] I am glad to see the corrective phrase. But this barely qualified relativism is similar to the "ethics" taught by Alex Comfort in *The Joy of Sex,*[4] one of the works Francoeur cites with approval. If he intends to do justice to a Christian doctrine of personal sin, Alex Comfort's teachings are a radically inadequate source.

Without joining the ranks of the frightened and ignorant who attribute AIDS to the wrath of God, we must be especially cautious, in the light of the AIDS event, about rose-tinted assessments of human nature. Here we are nose-to-nose with a disease causing death, a disease that forces us to reflect on our past and present sexual behavior. It would be worse than silly to ignore the shadow that has swept over recent discussions of sexuality. If Christian hope and joy are to be convincing in a context of such suffering, they must allow realistic room also for fear, pain, repentance, and forgiveness.

Precisely because sexuality is central to human life, Christians must acknowledge that sin affects our sexual relationships as it does the rest of our lives. People are especially vulnerable to the wounds inflicted in sexual relationships, and our anger and grief about such wounds sometimes prompt us to sin against those whom we want most to love. Thus, considered as sexual moral agents, we are both creative and destructive, both innocent and cruel. In precisely this area of life we need guidance and salvation from beyond our own resources. Christians claim that such help exists, that it is effective and available, and that it is especially intended for those—sinners and sinned against—who need it most. Indeed, the glory of Christian life comes not from our capacity for making ourselves new but from the knowledge that a new creation has already been begun in us. God's grace and love, not our own, are the warrants of Christian hope.

Francoeur focuses on images of human and cosmic play. As an archetype, "playfulness" belongs first of all to children; yet children can play safely only in a protected space. Christian sexual ethics must be protected by a reality whose scope is larger than the finite human subject. Human subjectivity did not make the world and will not survive it, except by the love and power of the One who did make it and loves it continually. Sexual ethics for Christians must be conceived and practiced in the care of that One.

But as soon as we give priority to God's love and power, we come back to the notion of a moral order whose integrity is guaranteed from outside ourselves, an order that undergirds our "rules of play." While avoiding the danger of ahistorical, abstract legalism, what rules can still be applied to Christians in our sexual lives? The best proposals I have seen for a "ruled" Christian ethics of sexuality combine at least two principles: autonomy and fidelity; universal respect for the human dignity of moral choice and a duty of fidelity in intimate relationships. The scriptural term that combines these principles is the word *covenant.* I would propose—with Margaret Farley,[5] Julia Gatta,[6] and others—that Christian sexual ethics include at its center the norm of "covenant" love between autonomous persons.

The two principles of autonomy and covenant fidelity, joined with knowledge of the natural range of sexual orientations, yield specific guidelines for Christian sexual ethics. First, if covenant fidelity is normative for heterosexual couples, it should be normative for every kind of sexual partnership. Second, if heterosexual couples are seen as "blessable" (i.e., as potential recipients of the blessing of God through sacramental symbols), then couples of every sexual orientation must be seen as equally "blessable." That covenants of lifelong, faithful, and monogamous love are not only possible but are already in practice among many lesbian and gay couples is evident. All that is lacking in such cases is the public symbolic witness by the people of God, and the legal and social protection and dignity that belong to married couples. Even without these supports, the quality of personal commitment shown by many gay and lesbian couples can be held up as an example of Christian fidelity.

Finally, I hope the norm of covenant fidelity can be applied in such a way as to entail no condemnation on those who are struggling toward deeper clarity and commitment and stability in their sexual relationships but who have not undertaken, or for some reason cannot undertake, a lifelong vow to each other. To say this is not to duck the meaning of the norm but to interpret it in a way that preserves respect for persons and honors the specificity of their circumstances.

A covenantal norm signifies a fullness of commitment, abundance of life, and totality of self-bestowal that *are possible in Christ.* It also represents a doctrine of love that agrees with psychological and moral experiences of deep commitment and a theological interpretation of the death and resurrection of Christ, which reveal God's love for humanity. Such a norm symbolically anticipates God's fulfillment of love, the great high marriage feast. A covenantal norm holds out a standard for human partners, a standard that should support people in their growth toward God, not punish their imperfect reflections of God's goodness.

References

1. There is also a second kind of subjectivism, which Francoeur's paper illustrates and applies in appropriate ways, a subjectivism based on experience. Like Francoeur, I think Christians should embrace the warrants of experience, including empirical science, as a factor in moral discourse. For example, much is known now, as Francoeur states, about prenatal and early postnatal influences on sexual orientation. We cannot pretend any longer that individuals freely "choose" their capacity to experience sexual love for people of one sex or the other.

2. As an antidote to authoritarian legalism, the turn to the subject is a time-honored move. It was this turn to the subject that helped Western religious thought escape its medieval servitude to an unchanging heaven and find its way to the lovely earth- and human-centered optimism of the Renaissance. Francoeur's opening quotation from Pico della Mirandola beautifully illustrates that shift to the subject. The Protestant Reformers' emphasis on personal faith, the Enlightenment's confidence in the natural reason of individuals, and still later the Romantics' claims for human creative genius all take subjectivity as their starting point.

3. Francoeur, "New Dimensions in Human Sexuality," p. 93; italics added.

4. A. Comfort, *The Joy of Sex* (New York: Crown, 1972).

5. Margaret A. Farley, *Personal Commitments: Beginning, Keeping, Changing* (San Francisco: Harper & Row, 1986); see especially the last chapter, titled "Commitment, Covenant, and Faith."

6. Julia Gatta, a priest in the Diocese of Connecticut, has written an excellent criticism of the "Report by the Task Force of the Diocese of Newark on Changing Patterns of Sexuality and Family Life" in a letter, dated March 24, 1987, to Bishop Arthur Walmsley. She kindly allowed me to see a copy of her letter, in which she stresses the standard of covenant for reasons similar to those given by Margaret Farley.

Biographical Note

Ann C. Lammers earned the degree of doctor of philosophy in theology/psychology/ethics at Yale University. Her dissertation was a study of theology and psychology: Victor White and C.G. Jung. She holds a theology degree from the General Theological Seminary and a baccalaureate degree from Barnard. She is assistant professor of theology and ethics at Church Divinity School of the Pacific.

Eros without *Thanatos*

A. Oliver Vannorsdall

Robert Francoeur has proposed "an outline for reexamining the Christian meaning of Creation and sexuality" utilizing excellent sources taken from the realms of process theology, phenomenology, sociology of religion, anthropology of religion, and contemporary humanistic thought. He has described very well "what is" in the realm of sexual practices and mores in our society as well as some of the contemporary and liberal theological response to these practices.

Although Francoeur has referred to the dichotomy within the human spirit resulting in estrangement from our true selves and others, he has overemphasized our "panerotic potential" at the expense of dealing with our finiteness, the dichotomies of our human nature,[1] and our movement toward death, especially with the impact of AIDS in our culture. Perhaps we need to explore even more deeply our "panerotic potential" for being open to Otherness, especially in the midst of pain, suffering, and death.

The AIDS crisis has brought our mortality out of hiding! This crisis has called into question our scientific, technological, capitalistic worldview in a way not made possible by the various movements of the sixties and seventies.[2]

Underneath our fear of failure lies the fear of death itself. Our fear of death has driven many in our culture—a culture that has stressed winning, victory, success, excellence, being number one, and being in control—to drugs and compulsive, addictive sexual behavior patterns. The New Testament's most powerful metaphor for sin is captivity to the fear of death (see Heb. 2:14–16).[3]

AIDS has brought into question the props provided by our scientific/technological worldview. Those affected often find their lives out of control as they are flooded with fears of the unknown, bodily disintegration, loss of family and friends. Often they are bodies motivated by fear without hope or reason, bodies separated from any saving word.[4]

Where do we look for this word? I do not believe that it is

107

enough to look at the enlightened literature on sexuality nor the pronouncements of churches at the national level, significant as they are. Taking seriously Francoeur's focus on Creation, we must look closely and listen to those he describes as ". . . cocreators who through faith, human experience, and risk strive to listen and respond to the challenges of a world and humanity moving toward the unfolding of the ultimate Kingdom." We must look to and listen to the struggles of those dealing with AIDS as they strive to deal with this illness. We must look to what meaning they have found and are finding if we are truly to be descriptive and experiential.[5] And we must not only look to see how they have found "pleasure" but to see their struggles for finding intimacy, commitment, love, concern, joy, honesty, trust, fidelity, transcendence—and, most of all, patience.[6]

I would suggest exploring more fully this concept of persons as cocreators (having the power to name) by focusing on Gen. 2:18–20. We are seen as talkers (*homo locquens*) and symbol mongers (*homo symbolificus*).[7] We are first of all a meaning-giving bodily being, a subjective-body that unconsciously intends itself. It is our bodily being-in-the-world, that prereflective level of our being, which can never be categorized, objectified, or analyzed, that is the foundation of philosophy, science, and language. This subject makes its environment by making it have meaning for itself. The body comes to orient itself in space (high, low), in the realm of sexuality, and other realms. The body seeks its way in the world, a body filled with "intentions," of our conscious and free life. The foundation of the individual is, not Descarte's "I think, therefore I am," but "I am able to."[8]

This body is not a thing but is able to take itself up in a transcending way. "The body, as a subject, is a self-transcending movement."[9] This existence, or power of self-transcendence, as giver of meaning, ". . . manifests itself in all human phenomena, in the gestures of our hands, the mimicry of our face, the smile of the child, the creation of the artist, speech and work."[10]

Ann and Barry Ulanov would call these forms of language primary speech or prayer. They write:

> Everybody prays. People pray whether or not they call it prayer. We pray every time we ask for help, understanding, or strength, in or out of religion. Then, who and what we are speak out of us whether we know it or not. Our movements, our stillness, the expressions on our

faces, our tone of voice, our actions, what we dream and day dream, as well as what we actually put into words say who and what we are.[11]

Response of the Church

The first response of the Church is to listen to the "confessions" of those persons confronted with the crisis of AIDS—their pain and suffering—as they seek meaning beyond the answers of our sedimented language and cultural systems and beyond their own shadow and counterfeit selves to become aware of what is best in us and what is worst. We need to listen to and observe their modes of language—their cries and laments, their desires, their aggression (anger), their fears, their projections, their fantasies, their sexuality, their praying for others, their gestures, their actions, especially their symbolic and ritual actions, and their attempts at creating community—their experiences of self-transcendence and otherness.

In my counseling I have listened to persons with AIDS (PWAs) and their loved ones talk of their hopes and fears and their desire and willingness to find meaning in the midst of loss, pain, suffering, and death itself. I have seen them move through their "I wants," their cries for security and affection, their "why me?" to a realization that what they want is beauty, truth, and love. They frequently find that in the otherness of those to whom they are attracted while seeking self-gratification and a cure for their loneliness, they are found by the Otherness of God. They frequently find this Otherness in death as friend, mother, and lover as well.[12] The Ulanovs write:

> It takes a remarkable kind of willingness to go with desire, to move with the feeling of the spirit, in order to enable one to experience this meeting with life at the source. Reality constantly discourages even approaching the possibility of the experience. The ordinary encounters of our world diminish desire by trivializing it, reducing it again and again to the most trifling stirrings and satisfactions of the flesh. Persons as persons are not involved in such exchanges, in which words, gestures, physical feelings, human concerns, and the postures of love are reduced to a mechanical enactment at the emotional level of a cigarette or candy vending machine. But even this kind of dwarfing of the large impulses of desire to the mechanics of sexual-

ity will not necessarily cut us off from the great presence that calls us. . . .[13]

The Church must be a voice that proclaims itself a community of persons willing to share and listen to others' experiences and perceptions of the world. The Church is that place where persons can lay before the Lord their desires, their anger and aggressions, their fears, their sexuality, their fantasies, their hopes and expectations. Here they can place before the Lord their attitudes and personalities—angry dependence, fear of failing, lives dominated by a myth of victimhood, lives dominated by a quest for power, lives dominated by a need for praise. We bring to the Lord's Table our experiences and perceptions and are given permission to do so. As the Ulanovs further write:

> God does not want the sacrifice that leads to death but living devotion, the sacrifice that leads to life, so that we give up into his hands all that identifies us, all the extremes of our being, our best and our worst. We offer our best love, our worst fear, our best wishes and hopes, our worst despair, our best values and our most corrupt, everything by which we have striven to live. We die to our own small versions of reality; we give into God's care our mythical gods and the gods of our personal and collective myths. These are the gifts we bring to our epiphany.[14]

In worship, Jesus' life becomes a model of one who fully participated in a finite world of evil, pain, and suffering—a person who faced these forces head on, a person who totally placed his fate in God's hands. Empowered by the Holy Spirit we are enabled to place more and more of our lives into God's hands as well. Through prayer and worship our lives are transformed and transfigured. In the realm of sexuality we can move beyond being in control or out of control to being under control; we can move from shame of our bodies and our sexual desires to acceptance and gratitude. We move from judging ourselves and/or trying to live by legalistic morality to living under grace. We experience that

> *Out of the turbulence of our lives*
> *a kingdom is coming*
> *is being shaped even now*
> *out of my slivers of loving,*
> *my bits of trusting,*

my springs of hoping,
my tootles of laughing,
my drips of crying
my smidgens of worshipping;
that out of my songs and struggles
out of my griefs and triumphs,
I am gathered up and saved,
for you are gracious beyond all telling of it.[15]

In the gospel we proclaim the life of Jesus who embodied fully what it means to be human. Here in the stories of the Bible, as well as in the lives of others in the community, we come to know God as Mother, as well as Father; to know God as servant and emptier of Self, who through her desire to relate and to be known gives of herself through the Spirit—that inner voice of compassion—confrontations and support that respond to our inner and outer "prayers" and whom we find to be in the End the sources of our innermost need to articulate, to find meaning.

O God,
I come to you now
as a child to my Mother,
  out of the cold which numbs
    into the warm who cares.
Listen to me inside,
under my words
  where the shivering is,
in the fears
  which freeze my living
in the angers
  which chafe my attending,
in the doubts
  which chill my hoping,
in the events
  which shrivel my thanking,
in the pretenses
  which stiffen my loving

Listen to me, Lord
as a Mother
  and hold me warm,
    and forgive me.

Soften my experiences,
into wisdom,
my pride
into acceptance,
my longing
into trust,
and soften me
into love
and to others
and to you.[16]

The primary purpose of the Church is the worship of God, as God is revealed in Jesus Christ. And its worship is eucharistic, for in the eucharist

> we engage ourselves in acting out a narrative which defines who we are in relation to God and each other and to the world. Our behavior in the Eucharist is voluntary, intentional, reflective, just, sharing, corporate, healthy, globally aware, forgiving and reconciling. And, in a curious way, it is political as well in that we give our consent to the ordering and leadership of our corporate worship. Our behavior in the Eucharist is not merely loving, it defines what loving is.[17]

In the eucharist the values related to love are acted out and are embodied in the ritual itself. They are not just pulled out of the air and applied to our embodied existence. We learn by doing and by playing.

> Worship is the most useless of all human enterprises, and consequently the most free. We do it because we choose to do it, not for any particular pay-off. Its results are unpredictable. It is full of surprises, although in its ritual it is and should be thoroughly predictable. Eucharistic worship permits us to enter a powerful vision of reality, the order behind the accidents where even pain and death become a part of human dignity subsumed in the glory of the eternal God. In the Eucharist our value simply as God's creatures, children, friends, is not questioned, but established and blessed. The Eucharist does not tell us what to do, it does not solve our problems. It simply lets us be, in time and out of time, what we were created to be.
> . . . How difficult it is to believe that we have a right

simply to be, to be here and now exactly as we are. The God of the New Testament revealed in Jesus Christ does not demand credentials or a resume. This God, a poor Jewish carpenter's son, the ruler of the universe, made us for himself. To be whole, to be healthy, to be saved, is to realize, whether we are sick or well, growing or dying, right or wrong, happy or full of anguish, that we belong at some deep, eternal level, to the God who made us, who suffered and died to bring us home. This is the most important thing about being human. This is the Good News.[18]

It is in worship and prayer that we are able to present to God our complete life, for

death is the act of freely presenting to God my complete life and the completed self I have constructed by every free choice I have ever made. . . . In shaping our world we are shaping our selves. God has given the human creature the incredible dignity of collaborating in its own creation, of being present at the moment of its own creation. God supplies only the raw material of existence (through creation), heredity (through evolution) and environment (through providence). These make me *what* I am, but *who* I am is up to me. The form I construct out of this matter, the statue I sculpt out of this marble, is mine and is me. Life is art . . . making—in fact self-making, self-creation. And the supreme act of self-creation is the act of dying.[19]

. . . in Christ God appears as our lover, who asks our free permission to impregnate us with His eternal life, and faith is our "yes" to that proposal.[20]

We structure (create) our lives by the stories (prayers) we express and through the rituals we create and in which we participate. We are truly embodied spirits. When we are placed on the edge, as we are with the AIDS crisis, we can discover new meanings, and we find that we are discovered by the Other who meets us there on the edge. Through a life of contemplative prayer we develop a contemplative availability to God, to the world, and to one another.[20] As we dwell in Christ through the Eucharist, we become what we eat, we receive who we are: the dwelling place of God; temples of the Holy Spirit.

References

1. "In the beginning was Alpha and the end is Omega, but somewhere between occurred Delta, which was nothing less that the arrival of man himself and his breakthrough into the daylight of language and consciousness and knowing, of happiness and sadness, of being with and being alone, of being right and being wrong, of being himself and being not himself, and of being at home and being a stranger" (W. Percy, "The Delta Factor," in *The Message in the Bottle* [New York: Farrar, Straus and Giroux, 1976], p. 3).

2. Excellent insights into the impact of AIDS on our culture are to be found in the work of John Snow, *Mortal Fear: Meditations on Death and AIDS* (Cambridge, Mass.: Cowley Publications, 1987).

3. An emphasis found in Snow's *Mortal Fear.*

4. A theme emphasized throughout Snow's *Mortal Fear.*

5. I think here especially of mothers who have lost their sons to AIDS. One of these mothers is Betty Clare Moffatt, author of *When Someone You Love Has AIDS.* Her sharing of her experiences during this crisis and her son's response to the crisis truly show that one can take ". . . the stones of tragic experience and turn . . . them into the bread of life, into nourishment and sustenance for ourselves and others." There are many other written narratives about persons dealing with AIDS, many of them revelations of God's grace working in the midst of death. I am reminded here of the writings of John Fortunato in his analysis of our culture in the light of AIDS in his book *AIDS: The Spiritual Dilemma* (San Francisco: Harper & Row, 1987).

6. This theme on the development of "patience" is to be found more fully developed in Snow, *Mortal Fear.*

7. Percy, "Delta Factor," p. 12. In his many novels, including *Love in the Ruins,* Percy has commented on the sedimented structures in our society. His characters are to be found moving in and out of the three stages of Kierkegaard. In his more philosophical writings, Percy could be characterized as a phenomenologist.

8. In this section I have taken many insights from the writings of Merleau-Ponty including *Signs* and *Phenomenology of Perception.* For more detailed discussions of Merleau-Ponty and Walker Percy see my article "Maurice Merleau-Ponty

and Walker Percy: Harbingers of New Age," in *Insofarforth: The Functions of Discourse in Science and Literature* (Papers from the National Endowment for the Humanities Summer Seminar for College Teachers presented at Michigan State University, Summer 1978).

9. R.C. Kwant, *The Phenomenological Philosophy of Merleau-Ponty,* Duquesne Studies, Philosophical Series 15 (1963), p. 48.

10. Kwant, *Phenomenological Philosophy,* p. 57.

11. A. and B. Ulanov, *Primary Speech: A Psychology of Prayer* (Atlanta: John Knox Press, 1982), p. 1. An excellent book of poetry that reflects the movement from the little things in life (a hug, a smile, a choice, a tear) to signs of the presence of the Kingdom has been written by Leo Booth, *Meditations for Compulsive People: God in the Odd* (Pompano Beach, Fla.: Health Communications, 1987).

12. See P.J. Kreeft, *Love Is Stronger Than Death* (New York: Harper & Row, 1979).

13. Ulanov, *Primary Speech,* p. 22.

14. Ibid., p. 122.

15. "I Praise You for What Is Yet to Be," author unknown.

16. "Listen to Me under My Words," author unknown.

17. Snow, *Mortal Fear,* pp. 29, 30.

18. Ibid., pp. 30, 31.

19. Kreeft, *Love Is Stronger Than Death,* p. 92. The use of sexual terms to discuss our meeting with God in death is also to be found in Dody H. Donnelly, *A Radical Love: An Approach to Sexual Spirituality* (Minneapolis: Winston Press, 1984).

The significance of prayer and the use of sexual imagery to discuss death are found in the following quotations from Kreeft, p. 105:

Prayer is incredibly simple. The only essential step is the first step, dying. Dying to myself and my world, giving up self and world and all the things self could be doing in the world instead of prayer, giving up the claim to ownership of self and world. . . .

Prayer is an affirmation of our creaturely role as feminine, as wooed, as impregnated, as responder to the divine initiative. Prayer is our response-ability, instead of our ability. We do not initiate prayer; God does. God continually proposes to us, "Will you be with Me Now?" And we usually respond, "No, I will be with myself; I will practice spiritual masturbation instead of spiritual intercourse." But when we weary of this emptiness, we turn ("repent," "con-vert") to God, and He fills us.

Prayer is the preparation for the last turning to God, for death. Perhaps everything that takes us out of ourselves is a preparation for death; love, music, and the honest pursuit of truth come to mind. But prayer is the best preparation for death because in it we are not only taken out of ourselves but also into the presence of God. Prayer is heaven on earth.

20. Kreeft, *Love Is Stronger Than Death*, p. 110.

Biographical Note

A. Oliver Vannorsdall is AIDS Chaplain at Parkland Memorial Hospital in Dallas. He earned the baccalaureate degree from DePauw University, the master's degree in sacred theology and doctor of philosophy at Boston University. He has been professor of religion at Nebraska Wesleyan University at Lincoln. Prior to assuming his position at Parkland Hospital, he served parishes in Houston and Lincoln.

Acknowledgment: I am indebted to Alan Jones for these concepts.

Part 4.
A Healing Ministry

Introduction: A Healing Ministry

For several years, now, whenever my adolescent son observes something he doesn't like or regards as repulsive, he states vehemently, "That's sick!" For most of my own life whenever I encounter something I find sensuously desireable I proclaim enthusiastically, "That's so good it must be sinful!" The words *sin* and *sickness* are laden with covert meanings. A discussion of them should be preceded by individual reflection on their connotations. That all parties become aware of these connotations and find a common basis for discussion is important.

Reader beware! Words have subtle power, with an unconscious impact on our souls. Words are eggs, with the potential of hatching and developing lives of their own.[1]

Lewis Carroll's classic *Alice Through the Looking Glass* is a serious book, a book of multiple dimensions. The claim by one of the characters that words mean whatever he wants them to mean is, I believe, a philosophy many of us practice. Let me put my cards on the table (eggs in the basket?): When I use the word *healing* I refer to a process of moving toward wholeness or oneness. Applied to an individual, I use it to refer to a unifying movement of mind, body, and soul; when I use it in an interpersonal sense, it means movement toward reconciliation where there has been estrangement; in a cosmic sense, I use it to mean moving toward becoming one with God.

When I use the word *cure* I refer to a remedy, a treatment of physical disease. Curing and healing for me are not synonymous. I have seen persons with AIDS (PWAs) healed before they died. They had experienced reconciliation with family and friends, and their souls were at one with God before the end of their lives. They died good deaths, in the Christian sense.

For Phyllis Leppert, sickness is an individual's perception of what is wrong with his or her life, and disease is an objectively measurable physical dysfunction. She and I are in accord as she speaks of "healthy dying." As a physician and as a Christian, she can speak of death as a function of being human. Healthy dying is an important aspect of our healing. She reminds us that we need to deal with our own mortality before we assist others who are dying. "To deny reality," she states, "is a sin. To face reality, to face ourselves and name what is really going on is to have healing."

Theology as Story

Health, health care, healing, the processes of disease, all are told in stories; in these stories, through interpretation, we can see God. A role of the Church is to interpret these human stories theologically and to draw out their implications, Robert Sevensky reminds us. Stories of PWAs can "become grist for a theological mill," he continues, "and there is a real danger of cheapening experiences. Bishop Borsch's comments on struggling with the naive natural law approach of many people . . . as not some kind of an abstract, academic, ecclesiastical cop-out but a real need we have [to see God in our experiences]. . . . People are by and large believers; there seems to be an innate need to make sense out of what's going on. This includes storytelling, the voice-giving aspect of religion. We need a theology of suffering which can see order where there is order and to help us endure disorder when that's all we can see."

How can we evoke theology from people's stories without imposing interpretations on them? One way is to interpret history, as William Doubleday interprets the cholera epidemic. Sevensky asks, "Is AIDS unique? What's special about it? In a sense it is not; it forces us to ask the same old questions and see whether or not the same old answers have any weight." He reminds us that our concern about the access to health care in the AIDS crisis can be applied to the other infectious diseases, to heart disease, to cancer. "We rightly focus on AIDS right now," he says, "but let's see it in the context of other diseases as well. Where do we allocate our health care dollars? AIDS is one of many issues in our culture and our theology."

Spiritual Healing

"What is the spiritual meaning of healing?" Sevensky asks. "I have reflected for years on what we do when we offer spiritual healing in our churches. We are giving voice to people; we are integrating people into themselves and increasing their immune response. Where is God in all of this? How does God act? It's an embarrassing question, but God is acting in this health crisis, God is healing in it." He tells us the English theologian Jim Cotter, in reflecting on the AIDS crisis, has stated that the goal of healing is the glorification of the universe.

Erwin Arriola: The Hispanic community keeps increasing in the Episcopal Church. Clergy don't want to know about AIDS. [They say that] it's not affecting our communities. And yet many of us working in pastoral care do it in secret ways since the beginning of the crisis. When I call people in New York [at the national offices of the Episcopal Church], they deny the reality of AIDS. It doesn't exist except only in the gay and white community. I am still being called, sometimes at three o'clock in the morning, when someone is dying in the hospital from the Spanish community, because we don't have a chaplaincy that is doing anything in our hospitals. You have to respond to the needs of our people. We don't have enough resources.

Electronic preachers are doing a great job in Latin America. They keep saying that AIDS is God's punishment. People believe them. The Church has a strong power voice. Whatever the Church says is OK. Our only hope now is that you people already working in the AIDS crisis, you that have the resources, will take a look into our community and start working together. Communication is the main key that is missing.

In New York [one-fifth] of the population [is] Hispanic. The [Centers for Disease Control] reported that two-fifths of the population reported with AIDS in New York City are Hispanics. How many people have died in silence, people that hasn't come out and say, "We are dying of AIDS," because it is God's punishment. Religion is important in our community. We have the power to tell the people, "It's OK; it's not God's punishment." They listen, but they still need to hear more.

One of the problems we face lately is the knowledge of the language and the background. [Cubans, Dominicans, Puerto Ricans, Brazilians: we have diverse backgrounds] but we do have something in common; it's our faith. It's not based in a biblical context, but it comes from the heart. We are discovering a new God; not a God of punishment that they taught us, but the God of Love that lives among us.

Health care in New York for the Spanish community does not exist. People is underpaid; most of them are illegal aliens; they have no access to medical care. Salaries are less than three dollars per hour if you are lucky, if you get a job.

Many of these people are drug abusers, bisexual men, gay men, and lesbians; but we don't exist, 'cause that is people that does not believe in God or wasn't created by God, according to many religions. Our faith comes from the heart. It is time for [the Episcopal Church] to start thinking in many different ways: first of all to get to know the language, the cultural background, and what is all the faith and religion that we have, and how it is expressed in a different way—and not only in a traditional theological context, 'cause our people is not educated this way. Our people, if they were lucky, they finish elementary school, and many of them only went to second grade. The American people are still expecting for our people to learn the language, to read material that has been printed for them in the white American way. Our people doesn't know how to read; our people needs new ways and different manners of education. We are trying not to take this white-oriented information, 'cause it's not working; it's just wasting money.

Health Care and Social Justice

"The health care system as it exists in America is absolute and completely bankrupt with respect to care for people who are poor. And it's getting worse, not better." This view of William Doubleday's is reinforced throughout the discussion. That view is particularly frightening to anyone aware that existing health care facilities are now strained beyond their capacities with the current population of PWAs and that the number of AIDS cases will continue to grow rapidly for the foreseeable future. A disastrous situation will only become far worse.

"I think that this problem has been around for a long time," opines Leppert. "It's just that HIV has brought it to the fore. Health care and research funds are given to the diseases that are the diseases of the very rich; there's a fancier cardiac cath lab probably in the hospitals in Fairfield County, Connecticut, than there are in AIDS beds in the city of New York. We are really in a tremendous crisis in the health care system. I really don't know what's going to happen. We are overwhelmed now. As physicians care for patients, we lose our colleagues and friends; we grieve; we are going through crisis also; it's very, very difficult."

Elizabeth Caton, a nurse living and working in Baltimore, tells a story that sets in bold relief the socioeconomic conditions in which technologically sophisticated health care may be provided in our culture. She describes a husband and wife living in the ghetto. The man had AIDS ("It doesn't matter how he has AIDS, because asking the question 'How did you get AIDS?' is a sick kind of voyeurism that allows us to blame something or someone.") The man was equipped with a Hickman catheter, attached to an IVAC pump, attached to a kangaroo pump, equipping the man to receive total parenteral nutrition through the night so that he is able to sleep without interruption for feeding. If he feels well, upon arising in the morning he may go to work. The visiting nurses had done an excellent job in training the wife to manage this technological gadgetry while maintaining sterility.

At three o'clock one morning Caton received a hysterical telephone call from the wife. The bed was wet. Her husband was bleeding. She didn't know what had happened, nor what to do. Caton rushed to the apartment and discovered that "a rat had come into the bedroom and chewed through the [intravenous] tubing. It was a very powerful image for me, about the kinds of realities that life in the ghetto, life in the barrio, life in poverty, brings. We can bring all this wonderful high technology to it, but there are certain realities there which daunt even the best of our technology."

Caton goes on to comment about Doubleday's statement that AIDS is a viral infection, not a moral infection. "I don't think that that lessens our responsibilities to be spiritual diagnosticians. My spiritual diagnosis of the problem of AIDS is one of loneliness; at the very bottom of this disease is loneliness—not just the loneliness that comes when one acquires AIDS. I think it may be the very cause or the impulse which drives us to those behaviors which try and dull the pain of that loneliness: to shove a needle in your vein for a momentary release of the pain of loneliness and isolation or to fill up that loneliness with lots of sexual relationships which leave us even more empty at the end.

"We can have all of the resources lined up, the high technology. But . . . we [must] begin to look at our churches as communities—and not as institutions of safety, of comfort, of a place to nuzzle up against the cosmic bosom of Mother Church and everybody get their share at that bosom—as a place where we really hear the call of Jesus to be community, to be a place where we can do the dyings and rebirthings that we need to do, so that our life can be celebrated in all of the manifestations and the epiphanies of that life. We had better be about the business of answering the question of Jesus, 'Who do men say that I am?' The way that we act that out is the real resource we need to take back to our communities.''

Addiction and Spirituality

"It's time to say to America that drug addition is to poor people in America what martinis are to Episcopal bishops and seminary professors," asserts Professor Doubleday, responding to descriptions of the inequities in health care. People treat drug addicts like trash. People of color do far worse with AIDS than white people. Women die much more quickly than men. But perhaps drug addicts with AIDS get the poorest treatment. Doubleday wants us to recognize that we are an addictive society. "It is the systemic sins of racism, poverty, economic and political injustice that have forced some of our people into drug abuse that is utterly dehumanizing. We can talk about AIDS until we are blue in the face; but if we don't deal with those more basic issues of racism, economic injustice, and addiction, in twenty years it will only get worse."

"About 90 percent of the population of this country is addicted," comments Fred Wolf, retired Bishop of Maine, now active in AIDS chaplaincy, "We know that for every active alcoholic at least six other people are affected and directly involved with the disease."

As in any crisis, the crisis of addiction offers opportunity. According to April Hockett, of the Episcopal Caring Response to AIDS in Washington, D.C., the recovery process provides an extraordinary form of healing in which Christ is present. She describes some interesting "crossovers" between the AIDS experience and recovery from addiction, and the "good news" of recovery as it relates to the Christian "good news." The spiritual issue of loneliness underlies both addiction and AIDS, and Hockett sees a search for transcendance in both experiences. For her, the recovery from addiction has been "more spiritual than the Church. When I told my priest that he said, 'Why do you think that's true?' I responded, 'The people in Alcoholics Anonymous know that spiritual development is a matter of life and death.' Christ is present in the pain of addiction. There is pain in addiction! Grace is present in the entry into recovery. Christ is present in recovery through the compassion in relationship to people in a tangible, personal way that I've not seen many people in churches able to do. Out of the desparation of addiction (which is seen as impurity by many people) comes a real desire for salvation, which, if the Church can speak to it, there are few things that are more powerful than that. Recovery is a conversion experience, a daily leap of faith.

"People are now talking about AIDS recovery. It is the recovering people with AIDS who seem to have what other people with AIDS want, spiritually. Why should this all be so difficult from the Church? We have a lot to learn from this. Our role is to enable grace, to embody the compassionate relationship, and to do all that through the Spirit working in us. I have been more blessed by recovering people and by people with AIDS than I have ever been blessed by the Church, and I'm a lifelong Episcopalian. I would like to find a way to let other people experience those blessings!"

Leppert cautions us regarding the concept of "AIDS recovery." People may recover from drug abuse, but they may have infected themselves with the AIDS virus. "Once the virus is in our body, it is there for life. I believe what we are seeing is people who are living with the infection, who have the infection arrested or are able to treat the opportunistic infections that occur. Perhaps we should talk more in the sense of the recovery as understanding our humanness. That recovery can mean accepting all of these things. We have to be very careful about the use of the term *recovery*. It is a different meaning. Not to do that is not to face reality."

Rosa Escobar: I am going to tell you a little story about a neighbor of mine, a young girl that was raised with my girls, that she became a drug addict and she became very sick and the family start to say that she have pneumonia. The little girl start to get skinny, skinny, and they are still saying the girls doesn't have AIDS when many people in our neighborhood know that's what happening. The girl was bring from one place to the other, from Haiti to Jamaica, from Santo Domingo to Puerto Rico, looking for all kind of help; but that doesn't work. By the time that girl was taken to the hospital, it was really too late.

Our hospitals! Our nurses and doctors are not ready yet to deal with the AIDS crisis. What they do with our AIDS patients is they are being thrown in a room. Maybe one healing person come around to take care of that person, but sometimes it is two, three, or four days that the persons is not being seen by the doctor. So the situation in the AIDS population in our community is a lot worse than the situation of the AIDS patients in other communities or ethnic groups. We mostly depend on Medicaid or Medicare. Sometimes, many times, these patients going into the hospital, and as soon as they reach the sixty days, period, on the Medicaid, they being sent home. By the time these people are out of the hospital they have no homes, no places to go.

About two weeks ago I have a person in my office that was thrown out of the hospital, and he have no shelter. He went to the shelter, but he was honest enough to tell the director of the shelter that he have AIDS, and he was told, "I'm sorry, but you cannot stay here." So he came to my office, and I send him to the other place, to the other hospital. He was kept there three days; three days later he was back. The question is that these people are being running from one place to the other, many times without having a hot meal in the day, running one hospital to the other, one office to the other, looking for help; but they don't have any help. I really believe that one of the resolutions that should come out of here today or tomorrow is to education our clergy, our lay staff of the churches. Because let me tell you there is nothing in the Bronx; just one meal program, and that's all we have there.

AIDS in the Global Village

"As a Christian, for the first time I cannot see any hope," a friend reluctantly acknowledged to Patricia Page, who has been doing research on Kaposi's Sarcoma in Zambia since 1976. Page directs our attention to the fact that AIDS is not only an international plague but is a relative newcomer to the United States. The virus ravaged Africa for nearly a decade on that continent, largely ignored, unnamed, and unheeded by the developed world. She recounts a conversation, on New Years Day 1985, with a friend who is head of the department of surgery in a teaching hospital in Lusaka. "It is probable that within the next fifteen years 50 percent of the population of that country between the ages of twenty and forty-five, people who live in the urban areas, the educated young people, will be dead. [The physicians responding to this crisis] have a simple test so they can vaguely figure out who is HIV positive; they have indication that 13 percent of the patients coming into an Anglican hospital in the rural area and 20 percent in the hospitals in the urban areas are HIV positive. There is no way to check the blood to know whether or not it is infected."

"In the government hospital in Lusaka," her friend reported, "we are not doing any surgery because we do not have oxygen and we do not have anesthesia." Page concludes, "My African friends are never well."

The Church as Health Care Agency

Ted Karpf pleads with the Church to recover our vocation as agents of health care, lamenting that we are estranged from those systems. "Our calling into health care was absolutely essential. Whether it was for five minutes in Zambia to be freed of the fears that are accompanying the loss of health, the loss of one's sense of being,—[this] actually gave one the luxury of talking about the relationship with a Higher Power. If we were prepossessed with simply trying to make do and even survive an illness, there was no opportunity for salvation. It simply was past the point of being able to be talked about."

Karpf then refers to a statement of Mohandas Gandhi: If God came to a hungry man in any form other than bread, that would be a travesty. He continued that "in the AIDS epidemic, if God comes to us in anything other than a recreated and a renewed health care system that allows a person living with AIDS to experience a moment of fearlessness to be able to deal with those ultimate issues, then we as a Church have failed grotesquely. There has been in our secularization a complete estrangement from the role of hospice/hospital and the role of health care."

Leppert, a Christian physician, responds. "Physicians are human beings," she reminds us, "and we have been as much a part of the culture that denied these issues as all [medical] lay people. We are troubled and searching for answers in a very profound and disturbing way. There is a place in the birth process called transition, which is exceedingly overpowering, where the contractions are so strong and so painful that it's almost too much. In a way, that's where we are now in the midst of this epidemic. We must get beyond it and come into a new era, a new birth. Physicians need as much compassion, caring, and understanding as anyone else. We have been somewhat arrogant in thinking we *did* have all the answers; we felt we could cure everything. We forgot to face the question of our need to 'heal' in the best sense of the word, in the sense of facing life and death and making life joyous. That's really what life is all about—it's what the birth process is about.''

The Ministry of the Laity

"The church does a lousy job of calling the people of God to accountability within the structures in which they work!" Tom Tull of the presiding bishop's AIDS task force decries. "The people of God are in the insurance industry that make the decisions [to cancel or not to cancel policies of PWAs]; they are in the [Food and Drug Administration]; they're in positions of power— we just elected one! [President Bush] is an Episcopalian. What we have talked about primarily are laity ministering in terms of pastoral care. The Church does a lousy job of calling the people of God to accountability for ministry within the secular structures of society in which they work—and not just doctors. What are the ethical issues involved? What does it mean for a manager who is a Christian to supervise subordinates? I never hear those issues talked about in my parish. We are not challenging our lay people, not holding up accountability; not supporting them in terms of making those difficult decisions about what it means to be a Christian in business and industry and in the [the government.] The Church is there making those decisions. There are Christians who are presidents, vice-presidents, CEOs, paper-pushers, in those organizations. The AIDS crisis presents us a lot of opportunities; one of them is to call the Church and its members to account [for decisions in the AIDS crisis]: you were there; you're the Church.''

"We have to realize that the ministry of the laity is not just passing the cup on Sunday or reading but that it is really being truly Christian and compassionate in the workplace,'' Leppert adds.

"A lot of our people have never heard of the baptismal vows,'' exclaims Doubleday. "I find myself preaching on them about three Sundays a month. Fortunately I move around a lot so the same people don't . . . [his remarks were interrupted with laughter]. But a lot of our people have never heard of them, and when they take a look at them they are rather startled. I fear they may drive the people out of the Church. The kind of seven-day-a-week committed Christian is inherent in those vows."

A Theology of Relationship

William Countryman helpfully points out that two topics are being discussed: the inequity of health care availability, and sin and sickness. He refers to the discussion of sexual ethics that is creating a good part of the Church's difficulties in dealing with AIDS. Sex always comes into the discussion of AIDS. He observed that "the renovation or recreation of our sexual ethic is a time-consuming task in itself, and it's also 'public health theology.' It really doesn't do anything for the sick person. Its goal is to create a climate in the community where people don't have to get sick in that particular way anymore. That's one reason the person sick with AIDS doesn't find it useful to talk about theology or ethics. What is going to be useful to that person is the kind of loving relationship that a chaplain or other caregiver/ friend/partner establishes with a person and the giving that takes place in that. We have already in our tradition the theological dimension of that available to us that has a function as critical theology—theology to apply to the critical moment: it is the good news about forgiveness."

Countryman continues, "The good news about forgiveness simply sets aside the issue of what your sins might have been, or my sins might have been, and says, 'God has forgiven us, whatever it was.' Sometimes we shy away from that because it gets applied in a destructive fashion by people who believe they don't have any sins, at least none worth speaking of, not which God would punish in any overt way. That's a perversion we cannot prevent; we will never have any control over the Jimmy Swaggerts of this world. What we can do is reassert the reality that forgiveness is either for everybody or it's for nobody. God on the cross does not say, 'You may be forgiven,' or 'You will be forgiven if you perform the following five steps in the correct order and really *feel* sorry in the process." None of that; the Christian system is forgiveness first, repentance second. You are forgiven first, then you can afford to repent. You can even afford to know what you have to repent of. That's probably scarier for the very religious than it is for anybody else; but that seems to me to be the way it works. That's a way of talking about the love of God that's being mirrored and conveyed in the love that's offered by the pastoral caregiver. It's theological language; it's language which enters into the psyche at the same level as all the theological stuff from childhood which said, 'You have been bad, and you're going to be punished now.' That's the level on which we have to work when we are dealing with the critical issue of people who are sick right now. That's every last one of us in some sense or other. Unless we see ourselves in the same category of people needing forgiveness and having received it, I don't see how we can ever speak good news to people with AIDS.''

References

1. ''Those of us who are workers of the word, by the word, for the word, and most importantly through the word, whether as analysts or patients, know what was meant when Oceanus told Prometheus: 'Words are the physician of the mind diseased.' . . . One of the names of God in Jewish tradition means quite literally: 'He who spoke and the world came into existence.' So, at the core of one of the most enduring mythologies of creation, the word is seed and gives birth to life and living things'' (R.A. Lockhart, *Words as Eggs: Psyche in Language and Clinic* [Dallas: Spring Publications, 1983], p. 85f.).

Sin and Sickness/Faith and Health

William A. Doubleday

> AIDS is a viral infection, not a moral one, and it is not
> meant to be a test of our personal hangups and moral
> beliefs. We minister because the person is ill through the
> activity of a deadly virus working its bodily havoc. . . . To
> argue that AIDS is God's punishment on homosexuals and
> others is illogical and morally repugnant.[1]

Since 1969 when Elisabeth Kubler-Ross wrote her landmark
study, *On Death and Dying,* a steady flow of books has told the
stories of people who have faced life-threatening illnesses.[2]
Frequently those individuals are heard to say, "Why me?" The
literature gives varied accounts of the helping professions' responses to that question. By contrast, the AIDS crisis has turned
the table. Now it is often not the sufferers of disease who are
heard asking a difficult and ultimately unanswerable question
but rather a lively chorus of judgmental clergy, unhelpful health
care workers, and opportunistic television evangelists who have
condemned people with AIDS with such messages as these:
"Why you? Because you are gay! Because you used drugs! Because you are a sinner! Because you are getting what you deserve! Because God is punishing you!"

William E. Amos, Jr., a Baptist minister from Florida, in his
useful book *When AIDS Comes to the Church,* observes that the
religious response to AIDS has tended to be based on either a
judgmental or an incarnational theological approach:

> Some ministers, in addressing both the issue of AIDS and
> the individuals infected with the virus, have responded
> from a viewpoint of *judgmental theology;* their state-
> ments have almost always included some clear words of
> judgment, spoken by the church on God's behalf, to those
> who are suffering with this disease. The presence of AIDS,
> both in society and in individuals, is seen as clear evi-
> dence of the wrathful judgment of God in reply to the
> behavior that caused the disease to be contracted. . . .
> There is a second approach, which can be identified as

coming from an *incarnational theology.*

> . . . An incarnational response centers on the people who are dying rather than on how they became ill. It struggles with a way to be present in their lives as the incarnate Word of God. An incarnational response understands the biblical reality that we are indeed our "brother's brother and our sister's sister" and their keeper as well.[3]

The "incarnational theology" described by Amos is, in fact, an authentically Anglican approach to the AIDS crisis. Indeed, many Anglicans, by virtue of our theological tradition, have responded to the AIDS crisis in a positive way in terms of pastoral care and with a prophetic voice in the public square.

For us, our faith is rooted in *Scripture,* and our knowledge of the Scriptures—our awareness of the substance of the gospel message—empowers the scope of our pastoral care. We know that in the Kingdom of God there are no throwaway people. We know that Jesus ministered to the outcasts of his day, even as we are called to minister to the outcasts of our own day.

Our faith is rooted in *tradition,* a tradition that believes in the healing power of the sacraments. Our tradition embraces human diversity and human freedom. Our tradition does not run away from controversial issues or from the need for a prophetic voice in troubled times.

Our faith is rooted in *reason.* We evaluate and employ the fruits of the labors of the human mind. For us, medicine, psychiatry, psychology, sociology, and anthropology are not demonic forces. Rather, they are gifts of God and tools for the pursuit of truth and caring love.

Our faith is rooted in *experience.* We try to comprehend beloved clergy and laity becoming sick and often dying from this dread disease. We are moved by men and women—sisters and brothers, parents and children, neighbors and parishioners—for whom AIDS is a personal issue and not just someone else's problem or presumed curse.

In contrast to the "Anglican approach," many of the more judgmental commentators on the AIDS crisis claim a "biblical view" of the epidemic. Emmanuel Dreuilhe, himself a person with AIDS, comments on this phenomenon in a chapter entitled

"Sans God, Sans Men" in his recent book on living with AIDS, *Mortal Embrace:*

> The hostility of religious leaders towards those who have AIDS poses an additional threat to patients who are believers: the preachers of the Moral Majority condemn them outright before millions of television viewers and call more or less openly for their destruction. . . . AIDS patients don't receive the moral support they're entitled to expect from their churches and particularly from the higher religious authorities, who maintain an attitude of prudent neutrality since they don't consider many AIDS victims to be good Christians deserving of God's mercy in their moment of trial.[4]

It is, in fact, very difficult to articulate a "biblical view" of AIDS or any other disease in the twentieth century in as much as our grasp of disease, science, medicine, and the human condition has changed so markedly since biblical times. As the German biblical scholars Klaus Seybold and Ulrich B. Mueller have written:

> One must first recognize that our understanding of the word "sick," of who is really sick, and what sickness really is, is to a large extent—and quite decisively—determined by the view of life and man our own age holds. . . . That means our understanding is relative, and that relativity emerges with a historical comparison.
>
> . . . one must remember that sickness is dependent upon the life situation itself; like all human things, it, too, has a history. Sicknesses emerge, proliferate, gain hold, and then die out.[5]

They observe also: "Sickness as punishment for past sins . . . easily seduces one into condemning the sick person and forgetting the necessary solidarity with the suffering."[6]

The AIDS epidemic is not the first time these issues have arisen. This point is well illustrated in the history of cholera epidemics in America. I am deeply indebted to Earl E. Shelp and Ronald H. Sunderland, whose absolutely splendid book, *AIDS and the Church,* first made me aware of the historical research of Charles E. Rosenberg published in 1962 as *The Cholera Years: The United States in 1832, 1849, and 1866.* Shelp and Sunderland summarize Rosenberg's findings:

> During the epidemic of 1832, cholera was said by many
> Americans to be a scourge of the sinful. "Respectable"
> people had little to fear. Only intemperate, dirty people
> whose behavior predisposed them to cholera were at risk.
> The perception of the link between moral judgment and
> vulnerability to disease reflected and reinforced prevailing
> patterns of thought. Cholera was viewed as a consequence
> of sin, an inevitable and inescapable judgment of God
> upon people who violated the laws of God. Cholera was
> not seen as a public health problem. It was an indication
> of God's displeasure with the people who contracted the
> disease.

> In the epidemic of 1849, the connection between dis-
> ease and vice still persisted. Also, the belief endured that
> disease is an expression of God's judgment upon persons
> and nations corrupted by materialism and sin. But unlike
> the cholera epidemic of 1832, the needs of people or-
> phaned or made destitute by the disease were not ignored
> by private charities and committees of "Christian gentle-
> men." Food, money, clothing, and other forms of assis-
> tance were collected and distributed. Some churches
> joined with these ad hoc committees of lay people, receiv-
> ing collections for the sick and impoverished. These com-
> passionate ministries were performed even though the
> victims of cholera were considered guilty of intemper-
> ance, gluttony, lechery, or alcoholism. The sickness or
> death of a so-called respectable person was considered
> anomalous and conveniently ignored.

> The nation's third epidemic of cholera, in 1866, was
> explained more in scientific than in moral terms. The
> theory that cholera was caused by a microorganism trans-
> mitted to the water supply in feces and vomit gained
> credibility but not full acceptance. Personal hygiene, sani-
> tation, disinfection, and quarantine became important
> ways to control the emerging epidemic. Prayer and fast-
> ing, stalwarts of previous battles against cholera, were re-
> lied upon less in an era of developing scientific knowl-
> edge and increased power to combat infection. Thus, as

physicians and public accepted an organic cause for cholera, the hand of God was no longer blamed and the belief
that moral failure predisposes people to disease lost influence.[7]

Of course, the equation of sickness and suffering with punishment and sinfulness did not begin with cholera. Considerable
scapegoating of sufferers of disease occurred with the medieval
plague and with other epidemics throughout Christian history.
The tendency to blame the victim can be seen in the experience
of biblical lepers and heard in the advice and opinions of Job's
so-called comforters. Actually, there appears to be substantial
biblical material on both sides of the sickness/sin dilemma.[8] But
when Jesus was asked directly about the relationship of sickness
and sin in the ninth chapter of John's Gospel, he does offer a
decisive response. Confronted with the case of a man born blind,
he is asked, "Who sinned? The man or his parents?" Jesus answers by saying, "It is not that this man or his parents sinned . . .
he was born blind so that God's power might be displayed in
curing him. While daylight lasts we must carry on the work of
him who sent me."[9] In the mind of Jesus, it would seem, the
focus is placed on healing and caring for all rather than on an
analysis of the sources of or reasons for sickness.

With that perspective in mind, I have confronted many judgmental health care workers and clergy, the sort who would say,
"The patients with AIDS don't deserve our care. God is punishing them. They brought it on themselves."[10]

As a chaplain, in order to combat these punitive attitudes, I
sometimes led surveys of hospital nursing units to analyze the
ostensible source of patients' illnesses. It was the rare patient
who had not in some way—to some degree—contributed to his
or her own unwellness. But only in the case of people with AIDS
did health care workers suggest that to neglect or stigmatize
patients was professional and ethical.

Clearly, blaming the victim is not good medical care or acceptable pastoral care. Indeed, the gospel mandate is to provide care
and compassion for all, no matter what the source of their
unwellness, no matter what our personal or religious views or
values, no matter what the source of their AIDS-related illness.

From another perspective on this same question I have often
asserted on the AIDS lecture circuit that an unduly anthropomor-
phic view of God sees a bearded gentleman on a throne scratch-

ing his head and asking himself: "Whom shall I zap today for their sinfulness? I know, let's give lung cancer to six smokers; let's give liver cancer to four alcohol abusers; let's give heart attacks to four people who consumed too much cholesterol; let's give colon cancer to two people who neglected to eat enough fiber; and let's give AIDS to eleven homosexual men and one newborn infant, and let's spare all the lesbians."

Looking at this issue from still another vantage point, the Right Reverend Paul Moore, Jr., Episcopal Bishop of New York, once observed, "If God is really punishing people with sickness for their sins, don't you think the perpetrators of war, terrorism, and nuclear destruction would at least get herpes?"[11]

Many theologians would argue that there are serious dangers in any religious view that is grounded in either self-righteousness or works righteousness. Most members of the Christian tradition have always maintained, "We are all sinners." There is alienation and brokenness in the lives of all. At times we all miss the mark of our finest and best potential. We are all participants in systemic sin, systemic sin that includes racism, sexism, economic injustice, bigotry, inhospitality, homophobia, and indifference. In fact, it is these systemic sins that compound the social circumstances in which the AIDS virus thrives.

Before proceeding to an exploration of some pastoral care issues related to the theme of faith and healing, I believe it would be helpful to recall where we may have come in terms of the complexity of the AIDS epidemic and its impact on people.

Early in the AIDS epidemic, most of us had a simplistic view of the illness and its sufferers. People with AIDS were branded as "victims." Treatment options were few and largely ineffectual. Long-term survivors were unknown. AFRAIDS (Acute Fear Regarding AIDS) was spreading even faster than the AIDS illness itself.[12] Initially, very few in the churches were concerned with pastoral care for those affected by AIDS. Those who ministered did so out of a strong sense of identification with the sufferers or tended to emphasize the care of the dying.

Perhaps the care of the dying was where the greatest need resided. Perhaps the larger picture of the epidemic and brighter hopes for those affected by the disease simply had not yet come into focus. Perhaps we were able to focus only on compassion for the dying because many were unable to seek acceptance or to offer care for those of the living whose life-styles the Church had neither welcomed nor condoned in the past.

But much has changed in the intervening years. Today, we hear many people talking about "living with AIDS"; we read about a growing number of long-term AIDS survivors; we learn how HIV infection may span many years of a lifetime.

Just as cancer is no longer accepted as an inevitable or immediate death sentence in our society, so too is AIDS becoming a challenge to battle; an occasion for healing; an invitation to explore or engage every spiritual resource that the Church, our culture, or any individual can muster into service. Clearly, to think of AIDS as a predictable set of symptoms, an inevitable course of illness, or an invariably rapid or certain cause of death is no longer sufficient.

Today, more than ever before, the AIDS epidemic raises a broad spectrum of life situations, including members of "high risk groups"; the "worried well"; people who are HIV antibody-positive; people with AIDS-related condition (ARC); the newly diagnosed; patients in an acute medical crisis because of some opportunistic infection; people who have been diagnosed for a while and are presently doing well and looking for resources for coping and healing; those whose bodies are seriously disfigured by lesions; those whose brain or central nervous systems have been seriously affected and who may be suffering from dementia; men and women wrestling with treatment options; those whose health is in serious decline; people who articulate the desire to "get ready to die"; those at any stage of the illness who are suicidal; people who experience a sudden surge of religiosity, perhaps in the context of what might be termed a "bargaining phase"; patients who must decide whether to forego life-sustaining treatment, such as going on a respirator; people wrestling with being discharged from a hospital, perhaps to die; patients who need a particular level of health care that is not available; those who, due to financial or insurance problems, cannot afford appropriate health care, treatment options, or life-enhancing drugs; people who are near the hour of death; those who are newly bereaved and also infected with the AIDS virus.

Simplistic stereotyping has sometimes caused us to miss the nuances and complexity of the AIDS illness as it impacts diverse and inevitably unique individuals. The predominant demographics of the epidemic in a particular part of the country, the makeup of our caseloads, and our ability to identify with certain of the so-called risk groups for AIDS will all contribute to our vision or blindness about who has AIDS, what their illness is like, and what their needs may be in terms of health care and pastoral care.

Social stigma, rejection by or alienation from family or friends, loss of job or housing or insurance, discrimination or neglect in the health care system, and rejection or denunciation by religious and pastoral leaders are not irrational fears but rather documented realities in the life experiences of many people with AIDS. These same issues, in varying degrees, also impact the families and the caregivers of people with AIDS.

Any consideration of the pastoral implications of the AIDS crisis should reflect upon the particular situation of the members of the diverse "risk groups." The following only begins to suggest the variety of life circumstances involved in the AIDS crisis: The homosexual or bisexual man for whom an AIDS diagnosis carries an implicit declaration about his life-style; the current or former drug abuser who has long been familiar with social isolation and rejection; those who struggled to leave drug use behind, only to be stricken years later by the AIDS virus; the hemophiliacs and transfusion recipients who have AIDS today because they followed their doctors' orders in the past; the grandparent who contracted AIDS after "successful" open-heart surgery or the school girl or boy who was infected by a transfusion necessitated by a childhood accident; women with AIDS—drug abusers, prostitutes, sexual partners of drug abusers or bisexual men—many of them people of color who already endure considerable poverty; women of childbearing age, some of whom will give birth to babies with HIV infection, while others will wrestle with decisions about terminating a pregnancy involving a fetus perhaps infected with the AIDS virus; prisoners across the nation, many with a history of drug abuse; a growing number of infants and small children—over 80 percent of whom are black or Hispanic—often with sick or dying mothers and in need of foster care; heterosexual contacts: the AIDS virus can indeed be spread by heterosexual means and in some urban centers a recognizable cluster of teenagers, college students, and young adults are already sick with AIDS.

In this essay it is impossible to give voice to all the diverse peoples affected by AIDS, but I quote from one of them with the hope that in our reflections we may hear a chorus of such voices. When I was the pastoral care coordinator for patients with AIDS at St. Luke's–Roosevelt Hospital in New York, I came to know a young man with AIDS who was paralyzed from the waist down as a result of neurologic complications. During his fifteen-month hospitalization—he had nowhere to go—he endured abuse and neglect by staff, great physical suffering, regular but often judgmental visits from family, and prolonged emotional and spiritual struggle. He was a spiritual seeker. Born a West Indian Anglican, he had in adulthood explored Christian Science, studied the Bahai faith, and for a while committed himself to the Black Muslim movement. His hospitalization in an Episcopal-related hospital cast him back into an Anglican sacramental faith that he readily embraced with strong encouragement from his mother. I visited him several times a week. At one point, a sense of hopelessness seemed to overwhelm him. In what now seems inspired pastoral desperation, I encouraged him to start writing a journal of his hospitalization. Much to my surprise a few days later he presented me with parts of a scrawled manuscript with the firm expectation that I would serve as his editor and typist. At the outset he entitled the document, "Waiting for a Miracle."

I read excerpts of "Waiting for a Miracle" at his requiem, but it has not seen publication. He, who must remain anonymous, began the account of his illness in this way:

> On wall number one hangs twenty to thirty greeting cards. Some were for my birthday, others are get-well cards, and the remaining few carried a note saying: "Hello! How are you? What is going on?" I feel I am blessed to have so many wonderful friends and I love to look at the cards because it reminds me that I am not alone.
>
> Now on wall number two is a large poster, Caribbean in feeling, with villages reminiscent of Jamaica or Trinidad. On top is written in bold letters: "There is no place like Home." This poster has brought me to many far away places and the dimensions of my limitating enclosure seemed to expand. Next to the poster is a picture of an elephant. For a seven year old, it is drawn quite well with eyebrows, tusks, and a trunk. My sweet little niece wrote

these words below it: "God Bless, God Bless You, Kisses from (Your Niece)." Each time I look at what my niece did I get a warm smile in my heart.

Wall number three is a picture of Jesus Christ. It is a good piece of art given to me by my friend Charles. It depicts Christ at the crucifixion. On Jesus' head is a crown of thorns. In the background is the cross. It is all done in pencil and charcoal. I've often identified with this picture. The suffering, his mystical depth, and his Semitic blackness projected many aspects of my self.

Lying in bed, wall number four I simply can't see.[13]

Like so many people with AIDS, he was well acquainted with the thought of suicide:

Several times I've heard voices saying, "Why don't you end all of this agony. Don't you know that it is unlikely for anyone to live more than five years with AIDS? You go get your nail file, cut your wrist, and in no time it will be over." Sometimes I wish I had a bottle of sleeping pills when I'll hear a voice. It is very soothing, caring, and full of authority. It grabs me tight as if I were falling off a bridge and says: "Are you crazy? Get those thoughts out of your head. Don't throw away your beautiful spirit and fall prey to Satan. Come to me, I'm your beloved. I'll take care of you. Have faith. Remember God will always be by your side. You'll be safe if you just learn to communicate with the Almighty."[14]

Over time he developed a rather steady spiritual routine that included communion on Sunday and pastoral visits by a team of chaplains, parish clergy, and seminarians. Of his own prayer life he wrote:

I've found you'll be safe if you allow God to come into your being. But I must be sure my spiritual communication system is working well. If I am really attuned correctly, I will reach God. It might be a voice. Often it won't be verbal, just a feeling of comfort and care. I pray every morning and every night. Prayer starts my day with grace and is full of optimism and hope. At night prayer makes my day complete. Afterwards I cuddle next to God, and lie waiting to enter the mystery of sleep and dreams.[15]

Very little of his account dwells on themes of sin and guilt. But there is one telling passage that describes a conversation fairly early in his illness with one of his "buddies" (friendly visitors) from the Gay Men's Health Crisis:

Steve, especially, helped me to know myself and to accept myself fully. He said: "You are not an oddity. You are just as much a man as anyone else. You have lots of talents and strengths to be proud of. Look at how many guys out there abuse their wives and children, are into drugs, mug, and do senseless killings. They are the ones who will suffer spiritually. But you love humanity. Look at how many friends are on your side and love you." "But Steve," I said, "I was wrong. I was promiscuous. I ought to be punished." He replied. "Do you know how many people out there are sick with AIDS and some don't even know they have it? Look at yourself. You are still alive and you are looking stronger and stronger each day."[16]

The last pages of the journal relate to the patient's experience of his own father's going home to die in Jamaica a few years previously. He closes with these observations:

The modern airport can be an unfeeling place to say good-bye. So we were all sitting in the waiting room. My mother, my sister, and I were all filled with grief. Finally the jet arrived. The stewardess came and put my father in a wheelchair. My mother stood beside him. My sister was crying intensely and she embraced my father and kissed him. I felt awkward. My father spoke my name. Immediately I hugged my father tight. My father patted me on the back and said: "Take care of your mother and your sister. Carry on, my son, carry on."

Through all the suffering and pain I've gone through, not knowing whether I would live or die, with paralysis, those words had an impact that give me courage and strength to overcome any affliction. *I will keep going and I will finally come to God. I will carry on.*[17]

He died a beloved child of the church into which he had been born, a few weeks after completing this last installment of his journal. I chose to include these rather lengthy journal excerpts because I believe that any discussion of the AIDS crisis and its pastoral and theological implications must comprehend the perspectives of people with AIDS. Likewise the perspectives of clergy, of physicians and health care workers, and of families, friends, and volunteers who have been involved directly in the care and support of people with AIDS must be heard with the utmost attentiveness.

The Reverend William Kirkpatrick, whom I quoted earlier, is an Anglican priest who has spearheaded AIDS ministry in London. He has written: "The ethical demand of our involvement in pastoral care is that of compassion. In the context of this ethic we must be aware of the dangers of drawing on theology to make quick and easy judgments. In so doing, we shall avoid the 'wrath of God' statements."[18]

For those moved to offer pastoral care to the sick, the dying, or the bereaved—or to those who care for them—there will always be the question of what does such care look like and by whom and with what values and attitudes is it *offered* and, *hopefully, not inflicted*. Problems often arise when religious groups, which take the position that they cannot and must not condone certain behaviors their tradition considers "immoral," nonetheless feel a strong scriptural mandate to carry out "works of mercy" for the sick, the suffering, and the dying. Often it is not clear whether such works are carried out for the sake of caring, as an exercise in pity, or for self-satisfaction. The nature of pastoral care inevitably also reflects the cultural and religious climate of particular institutions, communities, and regions. Even then individuals have great potential for help or harm. Several years ago, in an Episcopal-related hospital in New York City with an active AIDS chaplaincy program, it came to light that a non-Anglican staff chaplain began initial visits to people with AIDS by saying, "I am Chaplain X. You are very sick because God is punishing you. If you repent, you might get better. Otherwise you are going to die a miserable death. Would you like me to hear your confession now?"[19]

It is important to realize that every religious tradition—even the Anglican/Episcopalian one—has pastors, counselors, and chaplains who are able to minister with compassion and sensitivity, as well as those who will almost certainly deliver a message of guilt, judgment, or outright condemnation. Indeed, every member of the health care team may manifest values-based attitudes and behaviors that may interfere with the quality of care received by patients and their loved ones. *What is clear is that people who are sick, dying, or bereaved should be shielded as much as possible from proselytizing, judgmentalism, and intrusion on their privacy.*

The focus in AIDS pastoral care today must comprehend not only the issues of death and dying but the major themes of healing and coping. Most people with AIDS today choose quite intentionally to define themselves as "living with AIDS." A focus on living inevitably implies the need for resources for healing and coping.

In a scientifically sophisticated age, to focus on healing as a medical issue is perhaps tempting. To perceive coping as a psychological issue is perhaps even easier. In fact, the body/mind/spirit of the individual is so interwoven that such a compartmentalization of the human person—with AIDS or without—is far from helpful.

Recently, mostly out of the context of cancer care, a wide array of secular/nonreligious writers have raised the possibility that the individual's mind and mindset can and often do have much to do with the course and even the outcome of life-threatening illness. Norman Cousins has asserted the need for the patient to regain some sense of control and to maintain a sense of humor.[20] Carl and Stephanie Simonton led the way in popularizing the use of imagery in the healing and coping processes.[21] The New Haven–based surgeon, Bernie S. Siegel, M.D., has written *Love, Medicine & Miracles: Lessons Learned about Self-Healing from a Surgeon's Experience with Exceptional Patients,* a book that has become a virtual "bible" to some people with cancer or AIDS.[22] Louise Hay's books, tapes, and workshops are a focus for much positive healing energy in the midst of the AIDS crisis. Each of these approaches appears to have brought hope and resources for coping to individual people with AIDS and other diseases. Whether cures or remissions have been produced is at best a debatable issue. That these approaches have contributed to an enhanced sense of life for some sufferers is—at least anecdotally—a demonstrated fact.

Simultaneously, within the Church, pastors and writers as diverse as Morton Kelsey, John Sanford, Morris Maddocks, Francis MacNutt, and Kenneth L. Bakken and Kathleen H. Hofeller—to name but a few—have helped mainstream Christianity, including its Anglican branches, reclaim a vision and a role in the healing process.[23]

I see two principle hazards in these types of approach to healing, whether under a Christian or secular banner. There is often an implicit suggestion that the individual is, in fact, responsible for his or her illness. If such a suggestion simply feeds into and undergirds feelings of guilt, self-loathing, and depression, little good will result. If such a suggestion diminishes the fact that in the final analysis viruses and other organisms cause disease and in a relatively random fashion, again the individual sufferer may end up internalizing or self-directing negative feelings that might better be focused outward onto the causative organisms or elsewhere.

There is also a danger that the patients or patient families who embrace these approaches may be led to believe that they also control the outcome of the illness. If the patient gets worse or dies, they may conclude that they have failed, that they are responsible, that they have had insufficient faith, or even that God has singled them out for punishment.

Positive thinking, at least in its extreme forms, may be so death-denying as to become pathological. Some approaches to healing lose sight of death as a natural progression within life. Some proponents of healing ministries forget that in death itself we find healing. Indeed, in the nearer presence of God we Christians have long hoped to shed the hurts and pains of this earthly veil of tears.

Both psychological and spiritual approaches to healing may overlook the reality that a disease has a direction and course of its own. To argue that psychological or spiritual resources might at times delay that course and enhance the individual's perceived quality or actual quantity of life seems reasonable. That psychological or spiritual resources might ultimately change completely the outcome of a disease process seems more problematic; as yet I have seen no definitive scientific studies to document this possibility.

In the process of bringing pastoral care to people with AIDS, we have at our disposal within the Anglican sacramental tradition many resources for healing. Those resources are present in archetypal form in most services of public healing and in many other public and private liturgical observances.[24]

For some people with AIDS, participation in confession, whether corporately or privately, can assist in dealing with the sense of sin, guilt, alienation, and inadequacy they may be confronting in themselves. At times, repentance—surely defined quite apart from self-rejection—can be valuable in a new struggle with the AIDS virus. Sometimes wrestling with sin and guilt should be aided by pastoral counseling or psychotherapy, which are also avenues of God's healing grace. Sometimes the task for the person with AIDS is, in fact, to forgive the individuals who have caused him or her pain. So very many human ills of every kind are really the gaping wounds of past hurts and cherished animosities.

Holy Scripture, whenever read, not only recounts the story of salvation but also holds limitless potential for healing and enlightenment. In these days we especially need to read and reread Luke and Acts to encounter anew the central role of both healing and the pursuit of social justice in the ministry of Jesus and the early Church. Many people with AIDS have found particular stories and images with which they identify. I worked for many months with a patient for whom the parable of the prodigal son became virtually totemic.

As a pastor I have grown especially attached to the Psalms because in them virtually every human emotion can be shared with God, not just the pretty or polite emotions. I know too well that one of the most difficult human emotions is anger and that too many of us, including people with AIDS, are uncomfortable with anger, especially if the anger is directed toward God. Often we see anger toward God as a barrier to prayer and the religious life, when the Psalms demonstrate that anger may, in fact, provide a grounding of reality and strength to our prayer if only we will be open to its appropriate expression.

Prayer is an essential part of the armamentarium of Christian healing and pastoral care. Intercessory prayer is a ministry and discipline to which each of us is called. Our general and particular concerns for others in intercessory prayer help to bring God's healing love to bear on particular situations. The naming of names personalizes and grounds our prayers. But in the final analysis no prayer is complete that does not issue forth in loving care, social concern, and personal outreach to whatever extent is possible. To pray for people with AIDS is not enough if we exclude them from our fellowship and overlook the sociological factors that contribute to their plight. It is not enough to pray for people with AIDS if no one will visit them or advocate with them and for them in the church, in the health care system, and in the public square. The ministry of visitation in homes and hospitals by clergy and laity alike is both a mission to which each of us is called and the necessary embodiment of our intercessory prayers. Surely the high degree of participation by laity in AIDS-related volunteer and service programs is a heartening expression of this theme.

The laying-on-of-hands and the anointing with holy oil are two ancient expressions of healing purpose and intention within the Christian life. Their symbolic and sacramental power surpasses our understanding. Each represents a way in which we are touched by and marked for the experience of God's healing love. I will never forget one particular person with AIDS, long ago deeply alienated from fundamentalist Protestantism, who lingered for many weeks in a weakened and lethargic state. Each day I sat at the foot of his bed and gently touched his feet as I silently prayed. One day he raised himself up in the bed and exclaimed, "Are you doing the laying-on-of-hands with my feet?" That was the beginning of a new spiritual journey for both of us.

The exchange of the peace during the liturgy reminds us, people with AIDS and people without, that we need to touch and to be touched in our pursuit of health of body, mind, and spirit, and we are called to embrace and reach out to one another. Christianity is a communal religion. The gospel is a social message. In the final analysis, we must seek healing, not only for the individual, but healing for families, parishes, neighborhoods, and even for our whole church—our whole society. An essential part of the healing process is wrestling with those principalities and powers—with those systems, institutions, and policies—that stand in the way of health and opportunity for all of God's children. Pursuit of universal availability of health insurance and quality health care would seem to be logical expressions of this concept.

The eucharist—the Blessed Sacrament, the Holy Communion—represents God's most powerful healing gift to each of us. In it we are fed and nurtured; we are broken and made whole again; we are loved and healed. The breaking of the bread reminds us that in our brokenness we can yet find wholeness and in our woundedness we can yet bring healing care to another who is in need of love. Time and again I have witnessed the remarkable way in which the Sacrament of the Eucharist, whether received weekly or daily, brings the healing love, the nurturing food, the reconciling power of Jesus to the sick, the frightened, the forgotten, the dying, and the bereaved in the midst of the AIDS crisis.

If I were to summarize the faith that can guide in our pastoral response to the AIDS crisis, I would suggest these simple theological precepts:

God loves us. God embraces us. God reaches out to us. As his people we are called to do likewise: to love unconditionally; to embrace people with AIDS and their loved ones in their totality; to reach out with care and concern to even those people and groups that, in the past, we may have excluded from our care and worldview.

References

1. B. Kirkpatrick, *AIDS: Sharing the Pain* (London: Longman and Todd, 1988), pp. 84, 85.
2. E. Kubler-Ross, *On Death and Dying* (London: Tavistock, 1969). The literature inspired by her work is too extensive to detail here. See Therese A. Rando, *Grief, Dying, and Death: Clinical Intervention for Caregivers* (Champaign, Ill.: Research Press, 1984), for one of the better bibliographies on the subject.
3. Wm.E. Amos, Jr., *When AIDS Comes to the Church* (Philadelphia: Westminster Press, 1988), pp. 52, 53.
4. E. Dreuilhe, *Mortal Embrace,* trans. Linda Coverdale (New York: Hill and Wang, 1988), pp. 65–67.
5. K. Seybold and U.B. Mueller, *Sickness and Healing,* trans. D.W. Storr (Nashville: Abingdon Press, 1981), pp. 9–13.
6. Ibid., p. 189.
7. E.E. Shelp and R.H. Sunderland, *AIDS and the Church* (Philadelphia: Westminster Press, 1987), pp. 16, 17. Shelp and Sunderland summarize the work of C.E. Rosenberg, *The Cholera Years: The United States in 1832, 1849, and 1866* (Chicago: University of Chicago Press, 1962).
8. D.R. Bechtel, "The Bible and AIDS: An Example of Biblical Perspectives Informing Modern Theology and Ethics," in *Prism: A Theological Forum for the UCC* 12 (Spring 1987).
9. John 9:3,4, NEB.
10. Notes from the files of the Reverend William A. Doubleday.
11. Notes of a conversation about AIDS with the Right Reverend

Paul Moore, Jr., Bishop of New York, in the files of the
Reverend William A. Doubleday.

12. Editorial, Anonymous, *New Republic,* October 14,
1985.
13. Unpublished typed manuscript in the files of the Reverend William A. Doubleday.
14. Ibid.
15. Ibid.
16. Ibid.
17. Ibid.
18. Kirkpatrick, *AIDS,* p. 84.
19. Notes from the files of the Reverend William A. Doubleday, regarding interviews with patients and nurses.
20. N. Cousins, *The Healing Heart* (New York: Avon Books,
1983).
21. C. and S. Simonton, *Getting Well Again* (New York: J.B.
Tarcher, 1978).
22. B.S. Siegel, *Love, Medicine & Miracles* (New York:
Harper & Row, 1986).
23. M.T. Kelsey, *Psychology, Medicine & Christian Healing*
(San Francisco: Harper & Row, 1988); F. MacNutt, *Healing* (Notre Dame: Ave Maria Press, 1974); M. Maddocks,
The Christian Healing Ministry (London: SPCK, 1981);
J. Sanford, *Healing and Wholeness* (Ramsey, N.J.: Paulist Press, 1977); K.L. Bakken, and K.H. Hofeller, *The
Journey toward Wholeness: A Christ-Centered Approach to Health and Healing* (New York: Crossroads
Press, 1988).
24. My thinking about these resources was stimulated by
*Alternative Futures for Worship: Vol. 7, Anointing of
the Sick,* ed. Peter E. Fink, SJ (Collegeville, MN: Liturgical Press, 1987).

Biographical Note

William A. Doubleday has served time "in the trenches" in the
AIDS crisis, spending more than four years as the hospice chaplain at St. Luke's/Roosevelt Hospital Center in New York, ministering to persons with AIDS and their families. After completing
his undergraduate studies at Amherst, he earned his theological
degree at the Episcopal Divinity School in Cambridge, Massachu-

setts. He served a parish in Massachusetts prior to becoming chaplain to the Morningside House Nursing Home in the Bronx. He is currently director of field education and assistant professor of pastoral theology at the General Theological Seminary in New York.

A Theology of Suffering

Robert Sevensky

The AIDS epidemic presents in new and challenging ways perennial issues concerning the relationship of religion and medicine, health and healing. These include the complex of relationships between sin or immorality on the one hand and sickness and evil on the other.

Such connections come together for us in concrete ways in the AIDS epidemic. What is the relationship between sin or immorality and the particular instances of HIV infection, AIDS, or AIDS related complex (ARC)? What role does responsibility play, both individually and corporately, in the prevention, transmission, and treatment of these diseases? What is "natural" or "unnatural" about AIDS? What responses are appropriate and expected from those infected and those affected? What do faith and religion hold out in terms of health, healing, and ultimate salvation?

I will focus on three areas frequently overlooked in discussions of these issues. These include (1) the prevalence of faith and religious belief among the American population and the general effects these beliefs have on the experiences both of those who suffer from these diseases directly and those who perceive themselves as safe from infection and illness; (2) the question of responsibility for sickness and health and the ways in which this is confronted in the context of AIDS; and (3) the multiple and sometimes conflicting understandings of the connection between faith and healing and the mission of the Church to teach a more clearly balanced and nuanced approach to the phenomenon of spiritual healing.

Religious Faith: Its Prevalence and Possible Effects

In traditional and surprising ways, America remains a nation of religious believers. Over 90 percent of the adult population of the United States claims to believe in God; some two-thirds claim to believe in life after death; over half pray daily.[1]

These are impressive figures, even if we acknowledge that the content of terms such as *God* and *prayer* may vary widely from respondent to respondent and even if we recognize that for many people only fragments of beliefs from traditional religious systems remain, with much of the overarching framework weak or absent. They are important for appreciating the ways in which people encounter disease, sickness, suffering, and death. People do bring to these situations a whole catalog of views and interpretations, and prominent among them are religious interpretations, languages, and frameworks of understanding. This is true of people with AIDS no less than of others.

These religious and quasi-religious beliefs cover a variety of areas important in living with and making sense of illness, suffering, and mortality. As sociologist Peter Berger tells us:

> Every human society is, in the last resort, men banded together in the face of death. The power of religion depends, in the last resort, upon the credibility of the banners which it puts in the hands of men as they stand before death, or more accurately, as they walk, inevitably, toward it.[2]

What are these "banners"? I shall mention two.

The first is the voice-giving aspect of religion. Dorothee Soelle argues that one of the primary characteristics of suffering in any form is the reduction of those who suffer to muteness or speechlessness.[3] This is particularly true of suffering that, like that associated with AIDS, affects all dimensions of the human person: physical, psychological, social, spiritual. This is related to a syndrome of traits that *any* overwhelming threat to our integrity elicits: numbness, disbelief, isolation, turning in on oneself, helplessness, powerlessness, dependence, guilt, anger, despair, mental anguish, meaninglessness, confusion.

If this syndrome is to be confronted effectively, that is, if healing is to be possible in any sense, then voice must be given to the voiceless and a language to the speechless and the mute. Precisely here religion may make its most positive contribution: at its best religion provides the sufferer with a language to articulate his or her suffering and a place in which to speak that truth. Such expression—given in the language of the pastoral encounter, in the language of Scripture, in the language of prayer, in the ritual language of forgiveness, nourishment, and healing, in the nondiscursive symbols and symbolic acts of faith—makes possible that confrontation with proximate and ultimate reality that necessarily precedes both healing and change. This is the requisite first step in the development of sensitivity, rationality, and integrity, which are the building blocks of individual and social change. Likewise, if we are to integrate into our individual and common life those situations that cannot yet be changed or that are essentially unchangeable, then such expression is necessary.

The power of Christian healing services for those affected in any way by AIDS lies, in part, in this expressive function. Such services are frequently the only forums where we may express our anger and our grief. They are one of the few places where a language of suffering and of hope is given us, where honesty is encouraged, where companionship in affliction is publicly endorsed and effected. The services' healing power comes, at least in part, from their ability to allow those who are voiceless (and they are all of us!) to name our reality before God, ourselves, and others. They witness to an end to isolation, to the possibility and hope for human solidarity in changing the conditions that cause suffering, to the hope of divine cooperation in this process, and to a theology of suffering that can help us make sense of human pain without denying the reality either of that pain or of our outrage.

This theology of suffering can, at its best, help us to understand what is going on in our world and in ourselves, and it constitutes the second "banner" spoken of above. This need to make sense is primordial and pervasive. All of us seek to order and organize reality to reassure ourselves that things don't happen arbitrarily or by pure chance, that there is predictability, pattern, and rationality in what happens, even if such order includes a set of cosmic relations that occur randomly or are beyond our immediate control.

The approaches here are varied and include some understanding of the nature of created reality, its laws of cause and effect, and the way in which God, grace, or supernature relate to the Creation. It also includes the classic answers to the questions: Why? Why me? Why now?

The AIDS epidemic has forced us to reexamine our response to these questions. We have learned again that the question "Why?" is more often a plea for presence and compassion than an invitation for theology. We have learned again the dangers of the theory that teaches sickness to be the result of sin or immorality, to be directly or indirectly the punishment of God. We know what such a theory does to the sufferer and to our own vision of God and of the human community. We know, too, how other answers to the question "Why?"—it is a test, a purifying experience, a pedagogical device, a mystery to be borne sacrificially and in union with the redemptive actions of Christ—serve more our own need for order and explanation and less the needs of the afflicted. In the midst of this epidemic we must continue to be careful not to impose interpretations on those who suffer, thereby discrediting their own experience and the integrity of their own confusion or understanding.

At the same time, however, traditional interpretations have value for many today, and we must not be embarrassed when they are appropriated by those who suffer. The Church must continue to hold them out as possibilities for understanding and endurance.

The AIDS epidemic presents us with the opportunity and the task of rethinking our theology. There is something to be learned here from the purifying, testing, and sacrificial and redemptive suffering. In saying this we in no way need imply that God wills this disease and its toll. We imply, however, that nothing in Creation remains totally negative, that God will raise out of even these events a song of life.

As we know, God is already doing so: in the example of those living with AIDS courageously, graciously, powerfully; in the genesis of supportive communities of caregivers; in the responsible actions of many who are preventing further infection; in the frequently lonely voices of those in government who call for honesty over and against hypocrisy. There is a witness here to God and to the human spirit that must be held up for praise and for examination.

We must examine, too, our failure to respond, to be open individually, ecclesially, medically, and politically to those in need not only because of AIDS but also because of other life-threatening and life-diminishing conditions. We have been awakened by AIDS; we must not stop with AIDS.

Responsibility and Illness

A number of distinct debates occur under the category of responsibility.[4] There is, for example, the question of responsibility understood in terms of blame: Are persons with AIDS morally guilty? Are they morally responsible for their illness? Some have made distinctions between so-called innocent victims and those who might be termed "the guilty." Others have distinguished between those who were infected while they were ignorant of the causes and modes of transmission of AIDS and those who were afflicted through engaging in risky or unsafe behaviors after becoming aware of the disease, its modes of transmission, and methods of prevention.

There are important practical implications to such theoretical distinctions, implications having to do with the allocation of medical resources, with insurance coverage, and with funding research and treatment. The issues are complex, but if such distinctions are accepted as valid, a basic principle of justice applies: "Treat similar cases similarly. In this sense, AIDS is no different from many other (perhaps most) illnesses wherein human behavior wittingly or unwittingly plays a part. This is evident in the case of infectious disease; it is also obvious in such areas and behaviors as smoking, alcohol consumption, driving patterns, diet, exercise, stress, pollution, hazardous occupations and recreations, and so on. These relate in direct ways to cancer, heart attack, stroke, accident, mental distress, and a whole host of ailments, both physical and psychological.

The question of responsibility is not empty—we *can* affect our health. But such rhetoric must be applied fairly and across the board if applied at all. To only speak about AIDS and ignore the larger picture is dishonest in the extreme.

Another dangerous element implicit in the responsibility debate comes from exaggeration of the demand for responsibility into a metaphysical principle: We choose our own reality. This New Age doctrine takes a variety of forms: You got sick because your emotions are bottled up, because you want attention, because your life is out of balance, because your subtle forces or energies are deranged. The promise is also there: You can get better through emotional release, through laughter, through taking control of your life, through thinking positively, through a balanced or special diet, through imaging, through exercise, through meditation, etc.

There are peculiar difficulties with this strand of thought. On the one hand, there is a truth to many of these claims. There is an extraordinary complexity to the human person and much we do not know about the ways of healing. The human immune system is both subtle and responsive, and biochemical changes are certainly related to emotional, attitudinal, dietary, and behavioral factors. It would be surprising were it otherwise. Still, the claims of many of the so-called New Age healers clearly are overstated.

At their worst, these approaches reduce to a new form the ideology of victim blaming. Having chosen one's reality and having ignored the healing properties of the alternative system, those who fail to get better have only themselves to blame. Of course, these people may be ignorant of the healing power (of crystals, of herbs, or whatever), but in the final analysis they are responsible for both contracting their illness and for failing to get well. This is responsibility with a vengeance!

What shall the Church offer in the face of judgmental moralism? Among other things, we should offer (1) a doctrine of Creation that recognizes both the givenness and the essential goodness of Creation and of the natural structures while being open to their complexity and subtlety; (2) an understanding of human freedom that admits of degrees of freedom and responsibility and that acknowledges both the impossibility of absolute freedom and the very real possibility of lost freedom and the "servile will"; (3) a hope for human solidarity in the face of reality and for human cooperation in its amelioration, with structures that make such solidarity and cooperation more likely; (4) a hope for divine aid in this endeavor, not in the form of a *deus ex machina,* but in the guise of a rational theology of healing and prayer.

Faith and Healing

This leads directly to the question of the nature and role of spiritual healing, a complex topic due in part to the variety of meanings and expectations expressed under a common term. Martin Marty offers a helpful typology, however, in distinguishing four main clusters of beliefs concerning the nature of relationship between faith and healing.[5] These categories are by no means mutually exclusive; people can and do pick and choose among them according to their needs. Yet most people do generally fall into one of another of these groupings. I would paraphrase them as follows:

1. The "I am the master of my fate" position is naturalistic and materialistic in outlook and contains no reference to God or the supernatural; rather, it stresses human endeavor, natural process, and the Stoic virtues of heroic struggle, resignation, and self-transcendence.

2. The "I am in tune with the infinite" position emphasizes human cooperation with forces or powers that go beyond the empirically verifiable. These forces are inherent in the universe and are accessible to human beings, though they do not take the form of a personal God. There is a key to successful, healthy, and happy living, and that key rests in establishing harmony with both inner and outer forces and powers. The techniques to attain that harmony are seemingly endless.

3. The "God works a miracle in me" position stresses the direct intervention of a personal God in the healing process, one who, having founded the natural order, occasionally or regularly acts directly to change these conditions, thereby producing illness or causing recovery, often in response to prayer.

4. The "God experiences with me" stance tends to approach illness in natural terms but stresses both the wholistic nature of health (i.e., the interrelatedness of the various human dimensions) and the empathic presence of God in the process of human life, including the processes of sickness, suffering, and death. This empathic essence is generally viewed as working toward a final or transcendent wholeness that may include physical healing, but it is not limited to the physical. It may be combined with elements of (3) above, but it may well limit itself to the position that God's healing power comes only through the natural (if little understood) means of physical measures, psychological support, social involvement, and spiritual development.

While none of these positions in and of itself contradicts the Christian faith, some are certainly more useful in understanding what is going on when the Church claims to engage in a ministry of healing. I believe this is particularly true of the last position, which offers the basis for a uniquely Christian perspective.

The strength of this perspective lies in two elements. The first is the very idea of the empathic God. In the biblical portrait of Yahweh who feels with and for the chosen people and who works for their deliverance, and in the figure of Jesus especially, we are assured of a God who knows our plight because of sharing our pain. This is a God who is limited, yet limited not because of the nature of some intractable matter but because of the self-limitation that comes from giving a space for human freedom. Within those limitations, God works for the maturing, the wholeness of all Creation.

The other uniquely Christian quality results from the profound centrality of intercessory prayer in the Christian spiritual life.[6] In such prayer we pray to a God whose work in establishing wholeness is moved forward by our praying. God touches other's lives differently because of my prayers for them; by virtue of my reaching out in loving prayer to others, I am changed, and so is the entire divine/human constellation. Because of the empathic relationship established in both Creation and Incarnation, God can no longer be said to exist in isolation; God's very being is intimately bound up with ours, as are God's purposes. My prayers, by changing the context in which God acts, make a real difference in the healing intentions of God. In truth, my praying changes God! It is in this light that I understand the ministry of spiritual healing, that is, as a sacramental form of intercessory prayer.

Beyond this, the Church—that is to say, we—must abide in faithfulness, giving in neither to the temptation to flee the struggle nor to the lure of simple answers; doing what we can, supporting those who can do more, challenging those who do nothing; being really, if quietly, the Body of Christ in the world. This is a gospel ministry of healing for today.

References

1. See, e.g., G. Gallup, "Afterword: A Coming Religious Revival?" in J. Carroll et al., eds., *Religion in America: 1950 to the Present* (New York: Harper & Row, 1979), pp. 113–18.
2. P. Berger, *The Sacred Canopy* (New York: Doubleday, 1969).
3. D. Soelle, *Suffering,* trans. E.R. Kalin (Philadelphia: Fortress Press, 1975).
4. W. Wiest, "God's Punishment for Sin?" *Religious Education* 83 (Spring 1988), pp. 243–50.
5. M. Marty, "Religion and Healing: The Four Expectations," *Second Opinion* 7 (March 1988), pp. 61–80.
6. Adapted from a lecture on petitionary prayer by J. Empereur, SJ, delivered at the Graduate Theological Union, Berkeley, Calif., March 1980.

Biographical Note

Robert Sevensky, OHC, has been a monk of the Order of the Holy Cross since February 1986. He received the A.B. degree from the University of Scranton and the M.A. and Ph.D. in philosophy from Boston College, with a concentration in the philosophy of religion. From 1978 to 1985 he was assistant professor of humanities (religious studies) at the Pennsylvania State University College of Medicine. He currently resides at Holy Cross Monastery, West Park, New York.

Accepting Life Totally

Phyllis C. Leppert

I am here as a physician scientist, and it is in this capacity that I respond to the discussions on AIDS. Science provides us with the intellectual skills to search rigorously for objective truth. Ethical science appreciates at a very profound level that human beings see only in part; therefore, we must strive constantly for an open mind as we interpret observed phenomena, whether our perceptions are at the basic level of the molecule or at the level of interaction between persons, communities, or nations. In attempting to understand AIDS, we must continually keep open minds because the observations about this disease are changing at a rapid pace.

As a scientist I find it impossible to equate sin with sickness and faith with health as I define it. To the extent that faith, which encompasses a person's relationship with his or her God, contributes to a positive mental and emotional well-being, and that well-being allows for wholeness, it is possible to state that faith contributes to health. However, faith is not a necessary prerequisite for health. To the extent that sin separates one from God, that sense of incompleteness can contribute to physical sickness. Science has shown that chronic anxiety can depress the immune system to a degree. Physicians often make a distinction between *sickness* or *illness* and *disease.* The first two words mean that a person considers himself sick or that something is wrong with his life; the last word, *disease,* refers to a specific dysfunction of an organ or body system. People may shift between these categories. A person may feel sick and not have a disease. The reverse is also seen: a person can have a disease and feel well. Personal spiritual and religious beliefs are therefore involved in the sickness/health dichotomy.

In the long history of *homo sapiens,* other epidemics have had devastating personal, political, and economic consequences to those who survived them. The plague of the eleventh century is an example. Medical historians tell us that the spirochete responsible for syphilis was introduced into Europe and then spread through the world during the vast global explorations of that time. This sexually transmitted disease, which then had no cure, caused a terrible dementia, infected unborn children, and caused the death of kings and peasants alike. Society responded with fear and anxiety similar to our century's response to AIDS.

The AIDS epidemic involves two biological facts that invoke strong emotional responses in humans: death and sex. It is the complexity of the responses to these biological phenomena that produces the fears, anxieties, and ethical dilemmas surrounding infection with the human immunodeficiency virus (HIV) that causes AIDS. To confront them, we must confront death and our sexual nature.

Death, a biological fact, is an event all physicians face repeatedly in the course of their professional lives. Physicians turn, as others have, to poetry and literature to deal with this challenge. One has written this:

Another day—on call

The alarm sounds
another son rises
and begins rounds
sensing a hush
that has fallen
after last night's rain
through a misty calm
with blurry eyes
he passes the station
and hears the whispers
that tell
what he will find
when entering the room
the young man
with tears in his eyes
stands in a cloud
and he
his brother
lies silent.[1]

The silence of the cloud of death is the ultimate confrontation, so difficult to comprehend and to accept as a biological fact.

People often deal with death in an unhealthy way by using that most primitive and most entrenched defense mechanism: denial. Only by responding to our spiritual selves can humans come to terms with the reality of death.

The reality is that death, like birth, is constantly with us. Nothing will ever change these two biological facts of our humanness. With the advent of scientific medicine in the twentieth century, the death of a patient was perceived as the failure of the physician. A certain misreading and misunderstanding of science created a cultural arrogance that assumed the human species could control everything in the environment, including birth and death. Popular culture denied the reality that we are born *and* we die. Despite this attempted denial, it is clear from the biological perspective that to be human means to be born and to move toward death.

The spiritual, the emotional, and the intellectual quality of our lives depends on how we respond to these two fundamental biological points in the history of the individual. Our collective responses, our collective culture, including the institutional church, either add or detract from the quality of our collective spiritual journey, depending on the depth of understanding of our basic biological nature. We are born. We die. AIDS reminds us of these facts.

Ralph Crawshaw, M.D., has written a review of "The Phantom of the Opera." In analyzing the reason why this play is so popular, he writes,

> . . . the play unfolded as a full and complete metaphor, a modern morality play for the dread plague AIDS.

> Here lies the frightful moral of the tale. There is a dread phantom loose, not in our theaters, but in our culture, a phantom casting a curse on the most sacred belief of the twentieth century, sexual freedom. As a culture, we have rummaged around in our ancestor's attic and discovered that sexual continence, like a yellowed packet of love letters, is a man-made illusion, a family myth. We have discovered to our own satisfaction that the old constraints of sexual belief, of continence and commitment, simply no longer apply, for we have liberated ourselves from the ancient taboos of family life with our modern knowl-

edge—the biology of reproduction. For us, our modern belief systems are above reproach: we have science on our side.

Yet, there has proved to be more in that cultural attic than dusty myths. There is a presence there that now casts a spell over our vaunted belief in sexual freedom, and that presence is AIDS, an evil power that strikes with all the implausibility, unpredictability, and terror of the Phantom of the Opera.

. . . The Phantom of AIDS drives children from schools, doctors from patients, befuddles and confounds the brightest scientists, bringing to question all the certainty of our culture. Obscure obituaries report silent disappearances. Presidential commissions struggle with unanswerable questions. The press, in the emergency empowered as our educator, overflows with fatuous talk of new lifestyles. Our temples of healing, our hospitals, become death houses. In the presence of the phantom the richest of the rich are as helpless as the poorest of the poor. The contagion goes where it will, a ghost haunting laboratory and street. No one is safe; innocent children are born only to die. Our culture dances to a music not of our making or control, orchestrated by the unknown Phantom of AIDS.

What is our strength of mind, body, and belief against such an evil spirit that enters not just our culture, or our bodies, but, as the Phantom of the Opera, into our very cells, turning each body into an enemy against itself? . . . The fears of our childhood are the fears of all our life. We all remain children before the enigma of death. This is the ultimate family secret.[2]

The family he is discussing is obviously the Family of Man, our collective selves and not merely the nuclear family, a family that takes many forms in different cultures, including the gay culture. Both Family and family, however understood in a given situation, are important to the health of individuals. When this our Family, our support, is in disarray, we are lost; we are incomplete.

Our sexuality, another biological fact, links the fundamental points of our lives, birth and death, in a complex and powerful way. Not only does the sexual act allow for reproduction of ourselves, but at its best, in its joyousness, the physical act of sexual union produces a state in which we transcend ourselves and our mortality. The words we use to describe the emotions we feel toward our sexual love-object point to this. "He is divine," we say, or, "It was heaven." Words are inadequate to describe this physical act of coitus. At the climax we forget ourselves; we forget our humanness and the eventuality of our death.

In the human species, sexuality goes far beyond mere biological reproduction; it pervades our entire personalities. The outpouring of human desire can occur at any moment when sufficient stimulus, biological or psychogenic, is provided; that flood of desire, given the opportunity, can culminate in sexual intercourse. In most other species, the biology of physical readiness for the sexual act is linked closely to the ovulatory cycle in the female. The sexuality of human beings involves more than biology; it is also related to our perceptions. Our sexuality is more than physical; it is also emotional, intellectual, and spiritual.

How we behave sexually tells us about our acceptance of death. Obsessive sex often masks a fear of death. In classical psychoanalytic theory, sexual intercourse obliterates our unconscious knowledge of our eventual death. This psychological theory explains perhaps why AIDS, a sexually transmitted disease, is so terrifying to us. The sex act, which can make us feel that we will live forever, which makes us feel omnipotent, in the era of AIDS makes us confront the very thing we fear the most: death. In the age of AIDS, the sex act may lose its glamour, but we become more obsessed with sex. Sex becomes less glorious, less a mystery in the mythical sense.

This dynamic contributes to the hesitancy of the medical community (and from this, the hesitancy of the larger community) to name the epidemic appropriately. AIDS is a sexually transmitted disease and, like other sexually transmitted diseases, such as hepatitis, is transmitted by intimate contact with blood, semen, and other body secretions. Like other sexually transmitted diseases it can infect a fetus in the uterus. By not making these facts clear earlier in the epidemic, my profession contributed to the hysterical climate in our society, which was looking for scapegoats. In the United States we projected our fear of death onto groups in the United States that were infected with the virus first: homosexual men and intravenous drug abusers. These scapegoats were made the objects of our fears.

Intravenous drug use, leading to a fearful hell of an existence, spreads the virus and in some localities, such as New York City, is currently the leading risk factor noted in persons with AIDS. Because the behavior that placed these persons at risk may have occurred years previous to the onset of full-blown disease, many rehabilitated addicts are tragically infected. The obsessive use of drugs obliterates the fear of death in a manner similar to that of sexual intercourse. The drug high is perceived as glorious and has many physiological responses that are similar to the biology of sexual union. This, too, masks the fear of death.

Our biology provides a wide range of sexual expression under the control of the higher brain centers. These areas involve not only our emotions but also our intellect, in which lay our decision-making processes. In nonbiological terms, our sexual behavior falls under the control of our free will. Science demonstrates that the sexual orientation of humans, an aspect of one's sexual identity, distinct from sexual behavior, is a continuum from homosexuality through bisexuality to heterosexuality and is a complex biological phenomenon with many underlying facets. Science also demonstrates that within the framework of the continuum of the biology of sexual orientation, decisions regarding the actual behavior of an individual toward a loved person depend on the rational faculties. In other words, we are responsible for our behavior. The sexual drive is incredibly powerful and at its best is life-giving in the fullest; at its worst it produces the horror of child sexual abuse and the battering of a sexual partner. All physicians have seen this side of human sexuality. Sexually transmitted diseases are of the not-so-good part of our sexuality.

I believe the obligation and responsibility of the Christian community in the age of AIDS is to point the way to healthy sexuality, a sexuality that is not repressed, nor forced, nor compulsively acted out. The joy and play of healthy sexuality are glorious, and they do transcend death. Healthy sexuality in the age of AIDS means, among other things, avoiding infection. The dean of the Harvard School of Public Health reminds us that one failure is a failure for life.[3] The challenge to the Church is to understand the facts of AIDS without proposing a restrictive blaming theology. Christians know and need to bear witness to the truth that our sexuality is good and God-given.

The Christian community needs to be prepared to hear the dying person's expressions of regret over actions of the past. The most healing response is to accept these feelings of remorse and to then go forward and help the person forgive himself or herself, just as they are forgiven by God in Christ's death. The professional person, whether physician or priest, must be careful to avoid judgment; we dare not blame the victim, and we need above all to be compassionate. We also must be equally careful not to brush off statements of confession with platitudes. A person who states, "I was wrong; I was promiscuous," is entitled to have that statement accepted and then to experience forgiveness. Dying people do not deserve punishment. To discount the death-bed confession is an injustice to one's needs as much as blaming is an injustice. In the treatment process, the patient is entitled to feel the sense of his or her own guilt and remorse; these may lead to self-forgiveness. Only then does healing occur.[4]

We have discovered in the AIDS era that our actions and reactions make a real difference to our individual physical, mental, and spiritual health. John Vavra, M.D., has written a powerful essay in which he describes the impact on the living of their confrontation with death. He makes the point that we humans make our own hells. We have the power of rational choice against evil in whatever form it presents itself, whether it be a lack of integrity in our sexuality or a lack of integrity in the workplace. In examining my own life I have concluded that I must fight for change in the medical care system; for me not to do so would be to become enmeshed in evil.

Vavra goes on to say that great literature describing the confrontation with death "embraces the common elements of the description of life as a journey, the development of a new self-awareness arising as the result of a journey to the land of the dead or a descent into hell, and the termination of the journey in life renewal," as we allow transformation to occur in our lives.

When we exercise our wills in facing reality, we make choices. We then understand that the only way to face life is to confront the biology of life and the biological fact of death. In doing this, we then take another step in our spiritual journey. We develop new self-awareness and life renewal.[5]

The AIDS era has removed the veil from our own personal

sexuality, exposing our society's attitudes toward sexuality as well as its attitudes toward health and sickness. Our eyes have been opened to the fact that the health care system, as currently institutionalized in the United States, is a nonsystem, a monolithic bureaucracy that is sickness-oriented, not health-oriented, and cannot respond to a crisis. This system in the past did not respond appropriately to the swine flu epidemic that failed to develop, and has not responded appropriately to the AIDS epidemic. The AIDS epidemic, caused by a retrovirus originating in Africa, has stripped away our pretenses and demonstrated clearly that in the United States we spend more time, effort, and money on high-tech medical care of sick persons than on basic preventive education and health care. Our medical care system of uncoordinated federal and state agencies, community and teaching hospitals, and health centers affiliated with schools of medicine, have failed in the response to AIDS. I believe it is the responsibility and obligation of the Christian community to lead the way to a health care system that will serve all people, rich and poor, and at the same time be cost-effective.

Currently in the United States, HIV infection is spreading most rapidly through IV drug abuse in mostly poor minority communities. Minority women now contribute a disproportionate share of AIDS deaths. Like all diseases spread through blood and semen, the HIV crosses the placenta and infects the fetus. All babies born to infected, antibody-positive women will themselves have antibodies to the virus, but not all will be infected with the virus.[6] The rate at which infants are infected perinatally varies from 30 to 80 percent, but the average infection rate is probably about 50 percent. The overall health of the pregnant woman, as well as repeated exposure to HIV, seems to determine whether or not the fetus will become infected. The responsibility, therefore, of thinking Christians, I believe, is to make certain that the personal option of termination of pregnancy continues to be available to poor as well as wealthy women.

Another reality must be faced. AIDS affects us all: women, children, and men. In Africa, the majority of people with AIDS acquired the disease through heterosexual contact. AIDS is a disease of human beings, not just homosexual men. The issues around AIDS can no longer be linked exclusively with the issues of sexual orientation. The Christian community must make it clear that these issues are related but separate. Not to do so is a disservice to all persons with AIDS as well as to the homosexual and bisexual communities. AIDS has removed forever the veil shielding human sexuality from view in our society and has created an opportunity for the Church to study and to understand the sexual aspect of our humanness and the continuum of our sexual orientation. The Church must avoid illusion and understand the basic facts about the range of our healthy sexuality and the part that choice plays in this range of behavior. Only then can we promote responsible sexual behavior.

Also, church people must not continue the delusion of identifying a compassionate response to persons with AIDS with an understanding and acceptance of homosexuality. There is homophobia, and there is heterophobia, both equally misguided; the Christian community must understand that.

The questions raised by the AIDS experience go beyond these issues to the wider questions of health care, not only health care in the United States, but global health care: questions of how we as humans in all societies treat the dying, how we treat the poor, because AIDS affects the poor, both in the United States and other countries, especially in Africa, in greater proportion than the rich. We must wrestle with the wider issues of how we respond to and treat persons of color. AIDS raises issues involving the economics of health care, not only in terms of how we deliver this care, but also in terms of how we pay for care and basic scientific research. AIDS raises issues of caring and stewardship. These are the challenges that must be faced by our Church in the last years of our century if we are to be life renewing.

AIDS, perhaps even more than the nuclear threat, points to the need to promote worldwide peace and cooperation. If we spent as much on health as on armaments, would not the world be better? This represents the Church's ultimate and greatest challenge, and we must meet it. To avoid this issue is an illusion.

We need to put the AIDS epidemic into perspective. Persons die from causes other than AIDS; we must not neglect them. In Africa, more women are dying in childbirth than from AIDS. As Christians we must respond to this fact; we must also turn the real danger from the AIDS crisis into an opportunity to make a better world. The old Chinese proverb states that crisis is not only a danger but also an opportunity. To change things is in our power—if we only would.

Our faith offers us hope, the hope that comes with the acceptance of reality and the understanding that our intellect provides us with choices. We can make a difference. Our faith offers the hope that we are able to have the joy of life completely and honestly without illusions. We accept life totally. Out of this complete acceptance comes praise.

References

1. The author of this poem is Joseph R. Thurn, M.D., an infectious disease fellow at the University of Minnesota.
2. R. Crawshaw, "The Phantom of the Opera," *The Pharos* (Fall 1988): p. 37.
3. H.V. Fineburg, "Education of the Prevention of AIDS: Prospect and Obstacles," Roehrig, C. Burns, M.D., in *Science,* XXIX, #7(August, 1988): 592–97.
4. J.V. Becker, personal communication.
5. J.D. Vavra, "The Confrontation with Death," *The Pharos* (Summer 1988): pp. 16–25.
6. H. Minkoff, N. Deepak, R. Menez, and S. Fikrig, "Pregnancies resulting in infants with acquired immunodeficiency syndrome or AIDS-related complex: follow-up of mothers, children, and subsequently born siblings," *Journal of Obstetrics and Gynecology* 69(1988): p. 288.

Biographical Note

At the time she wrote this chapter, Phyllis C. Leppert was assistant professor in obstetrics, gynecology, and pediatrics at the College of Physicians and Surgeons of Columbia University. She was also a part of Columbia University's HIV Center for Behavior and Clinical Studies. During the first half of 1989, she served as visiting professor at the Tokyo College of Pharmacy. She is chair of obstetrics and gynecology at Rochester General Hospital and associate professor of obstetrics and gynecology at the University of Rochester. She earned her Ph.D. from the Graduate School of Arts and Sciences of that university, from which she also holds baccalaureate and master's degrees. Her medical degree is from Duke University School of Medicine. Dr. Leppert's professional career has been distinguished by numerous awards and memberships, and her publication credits include thirty-five scientific papers. She is an associate of the Order of St. Helena, a member of the AIDS Network of the Episcopal Diocese of New York, and has been a member of the vestry of Christ Church, Riverdale.

Part 5.
On Death and Loss

Introduction: On Death and Loss

"As a person with AIDS, I'm not afraid of dying," testifies Armando Rios. "Because of what I have gone through, I have learned that AIDS may kill me; it has been the most difficult journey of my life. At the same time it has been one of the most wonderful experiences for me, because it has taught me so much about being, or becoming, a human being and loving and caring. I don't know if I would have been able to learn that if I were to live fifty years and not have AIDS. The hardest thing with death and loss is when you lose so many people in such a short period of time; when you go to a funeral for a friend, and while you sit at that funeral, you find out that someone else passed away that same morning."

The AIDS crisis compels us to acknowledge that we all are dying; those with AIDS are simply dying faster than the rest of us. "The specter of AIDS catapults us into accelerated spiritual growth—or toward early death—and it all depends on the model of eschatological living we choose to follow."[1] The eschaton is the "last day" and eschatology is the study of the events of the end of time.

At the center of the issue of death is the meaning of one's life. The eschatological awareness that our lives are limited by time compels us to live intensely and in ways that are gratifying. The Apostle Paul lived in such awareness. The biblical writings of and about Paul abound with life-threatening incidents—natural calamities, accidents, political jeopardy—as he traveled around Italy, Spain, Turkey, and Palestine, by land and in little ships on stormy seas among the islands of the Mediterranean. He wrote of his attitude toward life and death:

> . . . with complete fearlessness I shall go on, so that now, as always, Christ will be glorified in my body, whether by my life or my death. Life to me, of course, is Christ, but then death would be a positive gain. On the other hand again, if to be alive in the body gives me an opportunity for fruitful work, I do not know which I should choose. I am caught in this dilemma: I want to be gone and to be with Christ, and this is by far the stronger desire—and yet

for your sake to stay alive in this body is a more urgent need. (Phil. 1:20–24, NJB)

It seems to me that Paul's attitude toward life and death provides a vital model for the Christian. It places the meaning of life in the context of the ultimate reality, which is God.

The literature of death and dying is abundant. The bibliography of this book includes works by Elisabeth Kubler-Ross, Derek Humphries, Edward Schneidemann, among many. The task at the Berkeley symposium was not to review the research data on death and dying and compare these findings with our own experience. Our task is to share our own stories. Rios spoke for many in his personal statement. The discussion of death and loss became, not surprisingly, the most intensive experience of the three days, and for many it became as intense an experience as any in their lives. Issues of the meaning of one's life, the reality of personal identity, the quality of relationships, and personal and cultural integrity intertwined themselves in the outpouring of personal sharing. That is the nature of the AIDS experience: intensive confrontation with one's self, one's relationship to God, and personal integrity.

Death and Passion

David Forbes, a staff member of the Bishop of California, comments on the sense of passion felt throughout the gathering and particularly on the passion "reeking" in the essay prepared by William Barcus (see "The Gospel Imperative"). "It is a passion that has to do with not one individual death or one person's loss to us but with that whole sense of death and loss tied up with the rejections our society imposes on the dispossessed," Forbes observes. Indeed, while our specific topic is AIDS, the broader and more universal theme is the marginalized people in our society, the dispossessed, and the "daily dying" that each person experiences in a society that treats certain people as though they are less than human or expendable.

> *Armando Rios:* Death in the Latin community is taboo. It's not something we like to talk about, especially if it's someone who has AIDS. It's automatically assumed that person is someone who was gay, and what usually happens is the family will not let the relatives or anyone else know that person died of AIDS—it would be something else: cancer,

diabetes, whatever. But it's not going to be the truth. The role of the Roman Catholic Church in our view of death has really done a number on the Latin community. It's not the same as we see it in the Episcopal Church. When someone has died of AIDS it's, "They have been punished." That is the main way of thinking in the Latin community. If you died of AIDS, it's because you are being punished.

How can we reach the Latin and black communities? When something is translated from English to Spanish, it cannot be done literally. One of the worst brochures I have ever seen for a Spanish-speaking support group said in Spanish: "Alone? Afraid? Do You Have AIDS?" Then it gave a telephone number. A person from a Latin background would not pick that brochure up from a table. That is culturally insensitive. We are not that open about what's going on with our bodies. When I discussed it with the person who made [the brochure], he said, "Well, they have to be Americanized." A translation must be done by someone who knows Spanish and is aware of the cultural differences in the language. [What is directed to the Mexican-American may not be suitable for Puerto Ricans or other Spanish-speaking cultures.]

How do you go about getting into the communities? Reaching the Latin communities will probably be through the women, rather than the men. The women are the head of the households; they are the ones who have to deal with everything at home. They are the ones who are the key to dealing with AIDS.

Death and Denial

Ted Karpf describes a conversation he had with his daughter Deborah, then a child of six, who for most of her short life was well acquainted with her father's ministry with PWAs. Deborah asked her father about a man of their acquaintance. In the midst of the conversation she stopped and very pointedly asked, "Daddy, does Don have AIDS?"

"Yes," her father answered. After a long silence, Deborah responded, "He was a very nice man, wasn't he, Dad?"

"He still is," her father replied. Then Deborah followed with, "I know, but it hurts too much when your friends die. He *was* a very nice man."

Deborah's healthy psychological defense mechanisms protected her against her hurt; to her, the friend was displaced out of her life summarily to enable her six-year-old psyche to survive. All too often many grown-up people use the same juvenile defense mechanisms long after the appropriate time in their own development to learn to cope more functionally with painful reality.

Karpf recounts the physical decline of a PWA in his parish, a man at the center of the life of the congregation, who sang in the choir and served at the altar. The blue and purple lesions of Kaposi's Sarcoma began to appear, his features became distorted, but he continued to worship and be active in the parish.

One Sunday several parishioners accosted Karpf and rebuked him: "The nerve of you, allowing [the PWA] to serve like that!" "It's one thing to talk about life and death; it's quite another to have it shoved in your face." "I came to worship God today, not to contemplate [the PWA's] death!" "I'm not coming to church any more; it's all too real." In their fear of death and unwillingness to confront their own mortality, they found it necessary to push their brother to the margins of their lives, to exile him from his own community. The truth that "in life we are in the midst of death" was not to be accepted and practiced.

Randy Frew of the presiding bishop's staff responded that he prefers to worship in a church where there is a prominent crucifix, vividly depicting the wounds and suffering of the dying Christ, as an intrusive reminder of the central theme of the Christian faith: the Incarnation (enfleshment) and the meaning of the death of Jesus.

Death and Confrontation with Reality

"We are going to experience some shocking parts of ourselves in either facing or denying the reality of the epidemic," Karpf warns us. "I think it is grotesquely unfair for any of us to speak to the Church about their involvement in the AIDS epidemic without understanding that the risk of that is going to break open in all kinds of places [as we confront] aspects of our lives that we may or may not wish to share in community." He then referred to the several comments during the weekend about the salvific benefits of Alcoholics Anonymous. In an AA meeting the story is the content. Everybody sits back and says, "That's my story, too." It's not merely in the telling of the story but in the identification with all the other story-tellers. However, in AA, death is not so immediate as it is with the AIDS epidemic.

The middle-American culture does not know how to grieve. On rare occasions we will allow ourselves physical, ecstatic grief. We allow our cultural inhibitions to deprive us of ecstatic grief (*ecstatic* means, in the Greek, "out of the standing state") that can provide a healthy expressing of intense feelings. How can we have the catharsis of experiencing the intensity of our loss—and then move on? In his parish, with all its AIDS deaths, Karpf reinstituted the old-fashioned wake, the dynamic party that was often marked by revelry and always by freely expressed feelings.

Earl Neil: In the black community, we do not deny the reality of death. In varying degrees we confront it every day, be it the nonphysical death, the psychological death in terms of struggling with our own identity and having persons recognize our identities on our terms; the death that comes from structural institutional violence in the political and educational systems; or the self-hate that is generated in the psyches of our young people. Look at all the gang violence and the fratricide going on down in Los Angeles, for instance; death to the human spirit. In different ways we are confronted with the reality of death. Basically, we are not afraid to "name this child" and to call death what it is. It is death; it is not "passing to the great beyond," or "hereafter." When you are dead, you are dead! That's real. But the reason we are able to deal with death and accept the reality of death is because we have an underlying commitment to life and to struggle, regardless of the vicissitudes and the violence and hate we have experienced from slavery on up through the present.

If you listen to the Negro spirituals and you hear, "O Mary, don't you weep, don't you mourn," there's just a vitality and a commitment to celebrating life and seeing death as a part of that; there is [a conviction] that there is life hereafter.

But also a part of the slave tradition, which comes from before black people were taken from the shores of Africa and brought to the West Indies or to this country, underlying that is the truth that African people are an emotional people. We sense a rhythm to life: the sun coming up and going down. We identified with nature and put it together by stretching out the skin from an animal slain for food over a hollowed-out log and then identified with nature by the beating of the drum. We are an emotional people, not afraid to express our emotions. Go into some of the Baptist churches, Methodist, Pentecostal churches in black communities, and you will see folk expressing their feelings. This whole relationship with nature that is not unique to Africans is that we saw ourselves as a part of nature and that we were not set on this earth to dominate nature, which European cultures did.

We even have difficulty with the Creation story in the Bible, when Adam is told to go and subdue the earth and name all the animals. When you can name something, you can control it. That has good and ill about it. You can name how to take care of the AIDS virus—medicine is built on that. When you can name something you can control it. With Africans and black Americans we never got into the great theological debates about the "is-ness of God." God is! God exists! When you can define God then you can box [God] in, as lots of European theologians did, and then [your attitude is], "Hey, God, you're this kind of a person," or "This part of my life can relate to that," or "I'll take care of myself."

We are an emotional people, and we are not afraid to express; so it's all right to grieve or cry openly in church or say "Amen." It's OK to show your grief because you know that is not the end of you! You know you're going to go on after that experience. You're not ashamed nor afraid of that, nor to risk being vulnerable, even among black Episcopalians. Blacks in the Episcopal Church bring something to it; it's a broadening of focus. This church has messed up the minds of black people, creating "Afro-Saxons" out of them! We have some teaching to do within our own black community in the Episcopal Church.

Contrast Neil's description of grief in the black community with the experience in the typical mortuary chapel that has an alcove off to one side, separated by a scrim, where "the family" can sit and weep unseen. It is assumed in the mainstream white American culture that something is wrong with visible grief; it is to be hidden and the grief stricken need to be protected from their emotional impulses. In fact, any psychotherapist can testify that grief is therapeutic; its effects are healing. Not to grieve, and to avoid having that grief witnessed, is frankly pathological. The bereft individual is helped when given an opportunity to tell the story and to experience its associated emotions. Supportive friends offer a gift of solace by listening actively to the story. When grief is suppressed or deferred, personal growth and emotional advancement are blocked, and the effects of the loss will be experienced at a later, often inappropriate, period in the person's life.

> *Erwin Rubiola:* In the Caribbean culture when someone passed away we have the mixture of African and Hispanics. [Armando Rios] mentioned something about rituals with music and stuff like this; it does happen. I experienced something like that in Central and South America. When it comes to grieving, at the funeral people will express their feelings; they will cry aloud, and it's the only time you will see the Spanish culture crying openly, too, and it's because macho [men] don't cry; crying is for women only. The Spanish community is still dealing with its grieving. This has told us also in the AIDS crisis that if we as Christians are to follow Jesus' teaching, our cross gets heavier, but we are dying slowly but surely in a different way. We are discovering a new God; it's not a God that will send you to hell; it's the God that comes and lifts you up, and that's the strength that our people is getting now; it's a new vision.

The Internal Auschwitz

One of the most powerful and transforming symbols of AIDS and those whose lives have been claimed by that virus is the Names Project quilt. The viewing of that quilt is an important source of the extraordinary stories developing in the AIDS experience. Edward Franks, a member of the presiding bishop's staff, describes his quilt experience: "I broke down, and all I could think about was, not the disease, but I had visions of

Auschwitz, of hate directed at the people who had died but then were told towards the end of their life that they were loved, [although they were] rejected while they were living. [Black] friends of mine . . . have said to me, 'Ed, I'm so tired of being reminded that I'm black. My color, which should have been recognized as a gift, has become a badge of hate by other people.' They have to live with a kind of 'Auschwitz' they've been given. Gay people have an 'Auschwitz' inside the head that they have to live with constantly. Other people have been given these 'Auschwitzes,' and it's the very same church that tells them they are loved that tells them they don't belong. It's funny that it creates a situation where you're living death before it happens physically. For me that was a kind of unveiling, and I had this vision of society creating these 'Auschwitzes' for people to embrace. I hope the church will come clean and try to do something about it, instead of giving us the cant it has always given that, 'we'll take care of you when the time comes, but while you are alive you can suffer all you need, and we will help you.'"

At the Foot of the Cross

How can we find the common ground between black, white, gay, straight, and Latino peoples? How can alienation and estrangement be overcome, the barriers between "the clean" and "the unclean" be broken down, and the oneness of God's people be realized in a visible way? Thad Bennett reminds us that "The common ground is, in reality, around the cross, around death and loss. Maybe that's the common ground to which AIDS brings us, that's going to break down even the racism of white gay men . . . [and] the distrust [to which Mwalimu Imara refers in his essay, "The Violated Stranger]. Maybe it's going to be at the cross where we may find our common ground, we may have the courage to meet 'the vital lie' [to which Ted Karpf refers in his essay by that name] and find out that it is a lie and to die to it! There we will not only find vital life but maybe even the resurrection."

Adds Earl A. Neil, M.S.W., of the presiding bishop's staff, "When I was in the fifth grade, I learned that in order to add fractions to make a whole number you must first reduce that fraction to its lowest terms, and then find the common denominator. Through the AIDS crisis we as people have been reduced to our lowest terms. Now we have to find the common denominator, and that common denominator for the Christian is Jesus,

who on the cross lifted us up above these divisions so we could
go on forward in his name!''

The Loss of Illusion

Normal human life is comprised of many, many losses, which
precipitate grieving to a greater or lesser extent. People often are
not conscious of their grief or do not identify it as such, and the
complex of emotional responses can then be confusing or even
denied. William Doubleday refers to these losses, sharing his
own learnings upon reflecting on issues of identity. ''I talked to a
number of people who shared a common theme: In coming to a
positive identity of one's self, one, in fact, must die to one's
illusory selves. In order to call one's self a gay person, one must
die to being the straight person you may have been taught or
your culture may have demanded that you be. In coming to be a
feminist, one must die to patriarchal values; in coming to be a
person of color, one must die to being an 'Afro-Saxon.' We all go
through stages and processes which, in fact, unite issues of identity with issues of death and grief. I have talked to many gay
people who can identify the time when they denied that that
was who they were, who had a period of anger, [who describe
engaging in] bargaining that involved playing the games that the
Church or society demanded; the periods of depression and real
sorrow and pain caused by the situation in which they found
themselves; and finally the experience of acceptance. The dying
in that circumstance is at least an echo of Good Friday, and the
new identity, the self-acceptance, is an Easter resurrection kind
of experience.''

Doubleday then points to an important task/opportunity, a
healing function for Christians to undertake in response to the
AIDS crisis: ''We really need to wrestle with those times when
the deaths which we endure do not produce resurrection experiences. It warms my heart when I hear about the persons with
AIDS who can identify their experience with AIDS as a life-
giving time and a resurrection experience. The fact is that's much
more common among persons with AIDS who are getting love
and care from all kinds of quarters, over against the persons with
AIDS who aren't experiencing anybody's care. Those people are
not sitting up in bed saying, 'This is the best time of my life!' Out
of death experiences can come life and resurrection!''

''As an abused child I had the experience of burying my true self," Ann Lammers shares, going on to amplify the concept of the multiple losses we experience in our lives. She explains, "It's too painful to have your true self attacked." She refers to the writing of W.E.B. DuBois in which he described the concept of black people having two souls: one that's really you, and one you bring out for show because it matches the dominant culture. Lammers summarizes the idea as it had been discussed in a group: "We described the marginalized people, [such as] women, laity, Native Americans. Some of the women in the group insisted that women in the Church have that experience. A couple of men in the group who were white said, 'It's hard for me to imagine anyone living like that.' Afterward another man in the group said, 'Wait a minute: I've just realized that was my experience; I was a child in an alcoholic family.' There is [a lot of] burying of the true self [in our culture]. We collude in burying the true self and keeping it buried. That means life isn't lived while we have the chance. Death is always going to come too soon if we haven't lived yet. That collusion with death is something we repent of . . . then we have to suffer through the grieving of everything we lose when we lay down the false self. If we can fight for the true self in the grief, at least we have the life we have; at least we have it while we are really alive: we are alive! People can actually come together, [overcoming estrangement and alienation] because they suddenly discovered they are alive."

Perhaps one of the reasons people are so frightened of death is the fact they haven't actually lived yet, and the life of the "false self" is hollow and empty. Death is feared because at an unconscious level one knows that she or he hasn't actually lived.

"It seems to me that any authentic encounter with death is a kind of surrender to truth," William Countryman emphasizes. "A surrender to truth is a surrender to God and a surrender to grace, and once you have surrendered to grace, as we learn over and over again in small ways and large, things are out of your hands. That's the only way resurrection can happen, because we can't produce it. Either God produces it or it doesn't happen."

Countryman shares a poem he wrote after visiting the Names Project quilt and the Vietnam Memorial in Washington. The poem concluded:

There is no life in us apart from theirs;

We are bound together, either side of death,
in this joyful, weeping communion.
Names, then be blest for your blest gift of tears
That giving love gives also rest from fears.

Reference

1. Howard Wells, a minister of the Metropolitan Community Church in San Francisco, who lives with AIDS, quoted in "We Are the Church Alive, the Church with AIDS," by Kittredge Cherry and James Mitulski in the *Christian Century,* January 27, 1988.

"The Vital Lie"
Ted Karpf

"In the midst of life we are in death." We are called to worship by these words from the Burial Office of the *Book of Common Prayer,* an office I have intoned more than sixty times for the members of my parish and have prayed silently as I have worked closely with another hundred or so of those within our city who have died from the consequences of AIDS. This anthem about life and death reminds us of the truth about living; namely, we are in death. In the daily reality of working with AIDS, we are perpetually reminded of our finitude and faithlessness as we confront the reality of death in our lives.

Death and "The Vital Lie"

While the recitation of numbers and the repetitiveness of the words tend to lead us to an intellectual assent to the reality of death—the reality of the physical end of our lives—because we are human, a special kind of denial of death is a fact of our lives. Because we are conscious about life outside ourselves and are symbol-creating, death is something more. Death is a force, a power that grasps the whole of our existence. In this way we talk about death in metaphorical language and with myth. The fear of death is no mere fear of physical ending; the fear of death begins in infancy and carries on through life in what Ernest Becker describes as "the vital lie." Becker quotes C.W. Wahl to emphasize this point:

> The child's concept of death is not a single thing, but it is rather a composite of mutually contradictory paradoxes. . . . Death itself is not only a state, but a complex symbol, the significance of which will vary from one person to another and from one culture to another. None escape the fear of personal death in either direct or symbolic form. Repression is . . . immediate and effective.[1]

This repression is characteristic of all human life. It is powerful and compelling, and, in the language of the Bible, is that which

185

St. Paul understands to be the nature of the power of sin over us. This force leads us into the vital lie of human existence, which Becker sums up this way:

> So one of the first things a child has to do is learn to abandon ecstasy, to do without awe, to leave fear and trembling behind. Only then can he act with certain oblivious self-confidence, when he has naturalized his world. We say naturalized but we mean unnaturalized, falsified, with the truth obscured, the despair of the human condition hidden, a despair that he glimpses in his night terrors and daytime phobias and neuroses. This despair he avoids by building defenses, and these defenses allow him to feel a basic sense of self-worth, or meaningfulness, of power. They allow him to feel that he controls his life and death, that he really does live and act as a willful and free individual, that he is somebody. . . . We called one's life style a vital lie; now we can understand why we said it was vital: it is a necessary and basic dishonesty about oneself and one's whole situation. We don't want to admit that we are fundamentally dishonest about reality, that we really do not control our own lives.[2]

Becker's words startle and disturb but do give us a clear and concise understanding of how death is as demonic as Paul has described it: "the last enemy."[3] Death is not demonic simply because it corrupts the body and destroys life but because it is continually present, perverting life into the vital lie. Life's energy is often spent in attempting to escape this reality as one abandons genuine human existence as intended by God. Death as reality does truly enslave humanity. It is power, force, slavery, chaos, terror. Death reveals our helplessness and uncovers our terror of nothingness. It unmasks our sense of meaninglessness and points to the abyss and chaos. When we begin our worship with the words, "In the midst of life, we are in death," we are striking a chord of fundamental and holy honesty and risking a confrontation with truth as we dare unmask the deception of the vital lie. Perhaps in this way the reality of AIDS is our meeting with ultimate reality, offering new possibilities for salvation, and life that is whole and full. Those of us who have worked daily with persons living with AIDS have seen nobility of spirit, courage of heart, power of the will, patience in the midst of suffering, and genuine holiness.

AIDS as Revelation

AIDS may well be the way for us to see the revelation of God, that is, the revealing of the truth about God and life in our time. For with the "me-centered," upward-mobility-seeking consciousness of those who live and swear by the vital lie in these last years of the twentieth century, AIDS cuts through to reveal us as a fearful, wanting, and needy people. AIDS is the contradiction of all that we claim to be true about our lives but reveals the most basic truth of being truly human and finite. Is it any wonder that all who suffer have been shunned by society, rejected in the name of fear, and have been forced to cower like animals? For the other reality of AIDS is that the longer one spends in the midst of the suffering, the more one comes to understand that to live wholly is to recognize that we are all persons living with AIDS. Some of us are the *infected,* but the rest of us are the *affected,* be it for good or for ill. To live without this recognition is to stand in judgment on all of life. Suddenly the distinctions between us are falling as we experience our common humanity, our common bonds created out of fear and hope.

In this bond of common humanity we are called upon to confess that the pain and recognition that come from a diagnosis of AIDS is real. We must face the fact that injustice—from discrimination against gay people to the rejection of the prostitute and the hopelessness of the IV drug abuser to the failure to protect our teenagers by sheltering them from the life-saving truth—is real. We must confess that tragedy is a part of life and not some alien form that has infused itself into life, and that tragedy is real.

But we must also embrace the truth that the courage of those who suffer and those who minister to them—the nobility of spirit to encounter death and triumph, the power of the will to survive against insurmountable odds, and the holy transformations wrought by love—is also real. AIDS is a signal and a reminder that the fullness of life is found in our movement toward vulnerability and away from the vital lie. In this cruciform expression of living, real life is found and is experienced as eternal. Perhaps only in this way may we proclaim, "O death, where is thy sting? O grave, where is thy victory?"[4] For in confronting the vital lie with the biblical revelation we are entering a perilous journey rife with possibility. While we may not be absolutely free from fear and death, we are embarking on our journey to freedom.

The Liturgy of Life

As we are ritual-, myth-, and symbol-making creatures by nature, the liturgical implications of embracing death as part of life are overpowering. We begin in baptism as those who are baptized into the death of Christ, which is to be baptized into the truth about life: namely, "nothing can separate you from the love of God in Jesus Christ." In the eucharist we break his body and pour out his blood and ours for a world in need of our intercession and ministry. As he is broken, so are we. But because he was, we shall never know the full devastation of utter desolation, because even hell has been redeemed by God. "By his stripes we are healed." In the sacraments of Holy Unction and Reconciliation we are given new possibilities to be healed and freed from our pain, our guilt, our regrets, our sorrow, and even our faithlessness. Holy Matrimony and Holy Unions, as well as Holy Confirmation, are signs that, while we accept the human condition, we are willing and hopeful in our making of commitments to honor, cherish, and serve.

Likewise the liturgical year reminds us of this confrontation of life and death and the meaning of being in the body. Perhaps most striking is the mystery and drama of our "Days of Awe," the days of Holy Week, as they lead us ever onward along a journey with Jesus from community to abandonment, from fullness to desolation, from dialogue to confrontation, and from pastoral care to prophetic action. In each form we see revealed the Way of the Cross as a way of living and being the truth. We experience, first hand, the mystery of incarnation and divinity so closely woven and delicately worn in the mantle of Jesus' nobility as he faces the temptations and trials of men and women caught in the web of the vital lie. We will experience no less in our own time, if only we have eyes to see, ears to hear, and hearts to perceive what is happening daily around us in the impoverished, oppressed, and afflicted. We see, perhaps all too well, that we are all of them, too, and that we are not free until they are free.

There is, perhaps, no other feast day that brings the tragedy of the human situation more clearly into focus than the Feast of the Holy Innocents on December 28. At the peak of our celebration of the incarnation of God we are abruptly reminded that we were bought with a price. The incarnation of God comes about in history and as such is subject to the price of our humanity and lack of it from the moment of birth. When facing those who live and die with AIDS, there is a great tendency to identify the transfusion recipients and the children and spouses of IV drug abusers or bisexual men as the innocents. But I say to you, everyone afflicted by this ghastly plague of death is an innocent.

As we face this tragedy with a sense of despair and hopelessness, it may be healthier to respond as the saints of ages past, of whom Jeremiah writes,

> *A voice is heard in Ramah,*
> *lamentation and bitter weeping.*
> *Rachel is weeping for her children;*
> *she refuses to be comforted for her children*
> *because they are not.*[5]

Part of our coming to terms with death and the threat of death is our refusal to be consoled, thereby dying we live. The poet Dylan Thomas summarizes this posture toward death in his immortal words,

> *Do not go gentle into that good night,*
> *Old age should burn and rave at close of day;*
> *Rage, rage against the dying of the light.*[6]

We must rage and live through it in order to find life. Our acceptance of death is not about going gently and peaceably; rather, it is about the acceptance of the reality of death as vital for lives lived with integrity, wholeness, and purpose.

Politics and Commitment

The political and social ramifications of the AIDS crisis are devastating. No longer can we as Christians, we who embrace the reality of death, stand idly by as the oppression of others continues. In so doing we are denying our part in others, our kinship with all humanity. No longer can we sit in silence as our brothers and sisters are denied adequate health care, reasonable shelter, acceptable nourishment, and needed assistance in order to live, nor can we blindly accept a national defense strategy that assumes "acceptable losses" in a nuclear holocaust that will kill tens of millions of persons. No life lost in the lust of war is an acceptable loss.

No longer can we elect officials who deny that something is wrong in a country that spends more on the care of household pets than it does on those addicted to mind-crippling, sensation-numbing drugs. No longer can we accept that while millions follow fad reducing diets, others are virtually starving to death at the back doors of gourmet restaurants. No longer can we accept that while millions die in Africa and Asia due to poverty, disease, starvation, and war, we stand by in our economic isolationist immunity as if it were nothing to us. Indeed, in the face of death and with the faith of the resurrection we are united in solidarity with all sisters and brothers in the name of all that is good and holy. Our denial of the reality of death is finally our denial of life. In such a denial we actually can believe that we are alone and immune from all that is life and reality. Perhaps the paradigm of a Lord who is executed for his own lack of immunity from these horrors is a paradigm for all of us today.

Living within the Rhythms of Life

To accept death as part of our reality we must learn to live within the rhythms of life, seeking balance and harmony with nature and finding our confidence in God. We must learn to live in the ebb and flow of the changes that exist between life and death, joy and sorrow, movement and stillness. In other words, we must forge a comprehensive vision of wholeness that is reality-based and faith-focused. This is no easy task for any one of us, as the culture conspires against us. Again this is where Paul understands and describes the corrupting power of sin as demonic; it is futile to go about attempting to preserve life: life simply cannot be preserved. The demonic power of spending all that we are and all that we have to maintain the fading blossom is born out of hopelessness and fear.

Compassion as Lifestyle

How, then, shall we live? The call of God in the time of AIDS is a call to compassion. Compassion is an active state of being present to those in need, often without answers or solutions. The pain of being present to another results from risking vulnerability and having the vital lie exposed within oneself. *Compas-*

sion is derived from the Latin words *pati* and *cum,* which mean "to suffer with." Therefore, the price of caring is entry into suffering with others as a way of living with others in this world. If we are caught by the vital lie, a life of "suffering with" is not a life we dare lead; but should we choose it we will discover a life that is filled by the very intimacy of our involvement with, and on behalf of, others. We share the story of our faith and faithlessness, and in us hope is reborn, love is renewed, and faith is restored.

The compassionate way is a way of movement, for in the throbbing, pulsing mystery of life there is a gentle movement from separation to union, loneliness to solitude, and from defensiveness to acceptance. The compassionate way, then, is a way of living that is life-affirming and accepting of personal differences and the uniqueness of others.

But nonmovement is stasis; and stasis—which suggests no change, no movement, no activity, no involvement—is death. Hence the compassionate life is a life lived to the full, regardless of risk, in which we discover our selves as we experience others. Compassion, then, is about being oneself without the blinders of the vital lie. While compassion makes us vulnerable, the paradox here is that we are then also living wholly.

For the person of compassion the question of the disciples to Jesus, "When did we see you, Lord?" seems ludicrous, yet holy.[7] Each of us will ask that question day in and day out, as did the righteous and unrighteous of the parable. The difference will be apparent when the righteous have done the deeds of charity, while the unrighteous will be searching for excuses as to why they did nothing. "Come, you blessed of my father" is the invitation to compassion and the call of all Christians.

"In the midst of life we are in death" is not only the call to worship but is also an invitation to life, a special kind of life, a life of compassion. In exposing the vital lie for what it is, we perform an act of exorcism, calling the demon by its name and casting it out. As we meet this demon in the AIDS epidemic, let us be aware that it not only resides in those who suffer and those who wish not to suffer but also in each and every one of us. To exorcise this demon takes the discipline of a soldier of Christ, the courage of a saint, the will of a martyr, and the peace of God. It is not a task that we enter into alone; rather, it must be within the context of community and in the humiliation of the Spirit, lest we confront evil and die. AIDS has revealed our darkest places of incompleteness and want. So be it. As these wounds are exposed to the light of Christ and the healing breath of the Holy Spirit, we shall experience the fullness of life as "dying, yet shall we live." Amen.

References

1. E. Becker, *The Denial of Death* (New York: Free Press, 1973), p. 55.
2. Ibid., p. 55.
3. See 1 Cor. 15:26.
4. 1 Cor. 15:55, AV.
5. Jer. 31:15, RSV.
6. D. Thomas, *The Collected Poems of Dylan Thomas* (New York: New Directions, 1957), p. 128.
7. See Matt. 25:37.

Biographical Note

Ted Karpf served four years as rector of St. Thomas the Apostle parish in Dallas. He earned the baccalaureate degree from Texas Wesleyan College and his theological degree from Boston University School of Theology. He has been very active in ministry to persons with AIDS as founder of the Dallas AIDS Interfaith Network; as cofounder of AIDS ARMS Network, a case management system; as cofounder of the Homeward Hospice; and as a charter member of Brian's Place Home for HIV-infected children. He is a member of the Dallas County AIDS Coordinating Committee and the National Episcopal AIDS Coalition.

Part 6.
A New Vision

Introduction: A New Vision

These words are being written in Advent, that time during the year when we stand with the threefold vision of retrospective, perspective, and prospective. In Advent we prepare for and refocus our understanding of history's most transformational event: the Incarnation.

In the age of AIDS, we have such retrospectives as Randy Shilts' gripping history of the deadly human immunodeficiency virus and the equally deadly political response by governmental, medical, and community officials.[1]

For current perspective, we have the stories shared with each other from our own experience and the rapidly developing networks, nationally and within local communities, such as the National Episcopal AIDS Coalition (NEAC). We have a keen awareness of the presence of God in our lives stemming from the AIDS experience, a strengthened faith, and a deepened spiritual awareness.

For prospective vision, we process the information gained and draw upon our understanding of ourselves as God's people and an awareness of God's will for us. We move ahead as people of faith, trusting in divine providence.

The number of people whose lives will be impacted by AIDS grows dramatically. It is likely that public health authorities underestimate that number. We urgently need preparation, of ourselves and the Church, for providing a ministry of healing presence among those whose lives are being disrupted by AIDS. We need preparation for calling the Church to a compassionate response, and for engaging society's institutions, compelling them to provide needed care in this crisis. A sense of impatience, invested with excitement, characterizes these discussions. The inaction of government and church during the decade of the eighties, while people grow ill and die, often abandoned and alone, is intolerable. We struggle for change.

The Challenge of Transformation

Gene Robinson's metaphor of the river is drawn upon and expanded, the metaphor that pictures a person standing secure on the river bank, hesitating before leaping into the river that represents change. The leap is risky, but transformation is not possible for those who cling to the riverbank.

In light of the fact that the language of Christianity is heavily colored with the imperative of change, that church people and institutions have such a reluctance to change is curious. We speak of conversion, repentance, renewal, reconciliation, amendment of life: to be a Christian is to be open to the transformations wrought by the power of the Holy Spirit.

Thad Bennett puts out these questions: "What are the things that keep you afloat in the stream? What are the pieces of driftwood that you have been able to hang onto in the midst of this raging stream? What transforms you so that you are able to keep going? Our belief is that those things that transform us, that keep us afloat, will be the things that transform the Church and will be part of our future visions and plans. Are there logjams in your lives that prevent you from staying afloat and moving with the stream?"

How do we summon up the courage to leap into the transformational river, trusting in the Holy Spirit to guide, comfort, strengthen, inform, and direct our lives into conformity with God's will? Ruth Black reminds us that we are already there: "At baptism we are hurled into the waters; we don't jump; we are already in there, and we are called again and again to see Christ in every person. [We must] find a healing within ourselves that allows us to deal with people [who are] vastly different, to love, [to] be angry as hell, but [also to] forgive."

The Christian Touchstone

Clearly, the baptismal vows, in which Christians commit themselves to seek and serve Christ in all persons and to strive for justice and peace among all people and respect the dignity of every human being, are the guiding principles among those ministering to people with AIDS. To attempt to be a Christian without recognizing this commitment is counterfeit spirituality, asserts Joel Mason, chair of the Task Force on AIDS of the Diocese of Atlanta. He finds counterfeit spirituality to be a logjam in the transformational river. "The HIV virus has revealed a sickness in the Church: the sickness of counterfeit spirituality. The only way to deal with that is to realize the baptismal covenant does not begin on page 303 in the *Book of Common Prayer;* it begins in our hearts."

"To stay afloat in the stream, we are called to be the stream, to be in community," suggests Edward Buckingham, an AIDS worker from the Diocese of Dallas, "We are that stream and we are in it to be the hands that beckon persons with AIDS to join us in that frightful place, to journey together, to keep our heads above water, to bind up all the wounds in the society, and we can only do it as individuals; but as individuals who are in community." His own parish, St. Thomas Church in Dallas, known for its ministry to persons with AIDS, "didn't welcome people with AIDS; we welcomed all people."

David Forbes quotes a character from Herman Hesse, Siddartha, who, while sitting by a stream heard a great chorus, not just the sound of the water but the sound of humanity. "The stream is humankind, not something out there into which we must plunge; it's something into which we swirl and are caught up, and in which we have our place. Who is this stream? The stream is a stream of hurting people, an image which returns us to the wounded Christ, who is indeed the metaphor of the Christ which must have meaning for me in the midst of this crisis." Forbes refers to a friend, in the final stages of AIDS, who is being tended to by hurting people. One is a man who is in the midst of a painful divorce. He also has a "telephone partner," a woman dying of cancer. "These hurting people are in the stream together because it helps." He has found his God in the midst of all the hurt. "We don't have to go out and invent a pastoral ministry; the pastoral ministry is in the stream; we simply need to get into it and raise our voices of hurt and praise and be as cogent and as expert as we can, but to be there and participate in that pastoral ministry that already is present."

There are many heros around us, both in the caregivers and in the PWAs. They often serve as "driftwood" in the stream, sources of flotation we can hang onto when the swimming efforts exhaust us. Pat Backman of Episcopal Social Services in San Diego tells us, "[The] pieces of driftwood I hang onto are the people I work with. They are a source of great strength to me. Our tradition of sacramental worship has been a great source of strength. The logjam for me is I do not have the strength to deal with the Church. I feel guilty about that when I . . . learn the whole purpose of this [discussion] is to deal with the Church. I can't do that right now."

"We are the Church," Ruth Black reminds us. "We continue to be only one person at a time plus the Holy Spirit; we can't forget that we are the people that transform; I can't change the whole hospital system, but I can change a few hearts in the places where I work. We are the Church, no matter how far we walk away."

Robert Brown describes the Church as "the world on the way into the Kingdom, being called into the life of God, in which we already live. As we work for a just society, we have an obligation as Christians to identify with those who are oppressed. All of us are called to identify with God's little ones. AIDS affects minorities who are traditionally oppressed people in our society: Intravenous drug users, prostitutes, gay men. The Anglican Communion is now predominantly people of color; I think the theological images of God and society and healing that come out of our broader community, particularly from Anglicans of color, will be crucial in determining how we respond responsibly to this crisis."

Dual Cultures

Perhaps each of the people participating in this weekend function arrive with (at least) two worldviews: Erwin Arriola, Rosa Escobar, and Armando Rios with one foot in Latin America and another in urban United States; Mwalimu Imara and Earl Neil with their roots in Africa and their ministry in America; the many with a life in the gay culture while being very present in mainstream culture. Christians, by definition, live in two worlds: the realm of God and the finite realm. The former has the view of death articulated in previous chapters; the mortal realm is terrified of death and exerts enormous energies avoiding and denying it.

"We are exploring, discovering two different roles needed by the Church," according to Albert Ogle. "One is the role of the shaman, or the mystic. The mystic is that person who is on a journey, going through deep, dark places to a place of death, [then] is resurrected to tell the story and interpret that story. Many of us know that story; that is who we are. The other role is that of the reconciler, a traditionally feminine role that holds together people who are diverse, or different, and today the Church needs that role."

The Spiritual Crisis

Repeatedly, those ministering to PWAs recognize that the AIDS crisis is essentially a spiritual crisis. Ogle admonishes us that "to maintain ourselves in the long haul, we have to dig deeply into the spiritual wells; we need to become men and women of prayer; take time away from the work to do the real work, which is spiritual; we need to feel centered and differentiated from the AIDS work. Spiritual nurture is vital."

"What AIDS has really done for me is make me a man of prayer" Gerald Anderson, of the Episcopal Caring Response to AIDS, confesses, "I am overwhelmed with the sense of what I haven't done as a priest. I certainly have prayed, but prayer has not had the power for me that it does of late. It has something to do with the sense of being connected with those who have gone on but also the sense of God's presence here, now, around us, in us, which I am really experiencing as a power like I have never experienced before. I feel like I am in the river; that sense of God's incredible power through others and through him/herself, and that connectedness, is what is sustaining me; it is what others are asking for. We have tremendous opportunity to witness to those who are coming to us, seeking answers."

The fearfulness with which church people (as well as secular people) respond to AIDS causes a great deal of concern. Marian Stinson, a clinical social worker from the Diocese of Los Angeles, preparing for holy orders at Church Divinity School of the Pacific, observes, "There is very little difference between having AIDS and the fear of AIDS. Both have to do with inadequate defense systems. One will kill your body; the other will strangle your heart and soul." Our task is to persuade church people that their fear of AIDS threatens to strangle their hearts and souls! God is in the AIDS experience, bringing about transformation and reconciliation.

The mandate for AIDS ministry is found in Christ, declares Edward Garrett. The early months of his AIDS ministry were performed out of an intellectual commitment. Then, as he gained more "hands on" experience with PWAs, he recognized, "The compassion of our Lord Jesus Christ is the ultimate authority of the Church. Through [my AIDS ministry] I've learned to cry. I've learned so much of rejection and hurt. It has broken through my eastern Ivy League facade.''

''We are transformation; we represent in our lives that which is going to transform—and is transforming the Church and the world,'' proclaims Ogle. ''Whatever is keeping us faithful is crucial to the exploration of thoughts and values that this dialogue is about. We represent two different worlds; we stand looking both at the old and the future. Many people in the Church don't have that vision of the future yet. Our greatest challenge is to interpret and convey to the Church part of that vision.''

Reference

1. R. Shilts, *And The Band Played On* (New York: St. Martin's Press, 1987).

Transformation: Visions and Plans

Albert J. Ogle

My aunt showed me a suitcase, empty, uninteresting. She then closed it and suggested that if I opened it again, I would find something inside it. With four-year-old contempt, I humoured her, only to find inside a string of pearls which she had bought for me.[1]

One of humankind's most primitive and timeless expressions is to mark important places with stones. In the wastelands of Ireland and Scotland they were sometimes known as "cairns," often marking important burial grounds and sacred places or orienting travelers. As a symbol I have found cairns a useful metaphor to describe both the contributions we are all making to the world as a result of an involvement with AIDS and to memorialize the events and people that called us into this journey together. According to a modern custom in some remote places, travelers pick up a stone and add it to a pile of marker stones also known as a cairn. These cairns can be helpful to future travelers where there isn't a clearly defined road. In the AIDS experience, there is no clearly defined road, but we know others have gone before us with similar, if not worse, anguish and experiences in their hearts.

Our transformation, then, upon which this chapter is based, is only of the cairns along the well-trodden path; we bring our few stones to the pile as memorials of the people and lives and events that have shaped ours, to be noted by those who come after us. Jacob built a cairn to mark the place of his encounter with God in that border country between the life he had known and the life of his uncertain future. The cairn marked a recognition of the beyondness in being apprehended by God.

Brian Urquehard, a colleague of Dag Hammarskjöld at the United Nations, once wrote in the *New Yorker* magazine, "Musing on the image, a friend writes of such cairns as substantial, designed, built, sharing in the environment, modest, unpretentious and very real waymarkers, recording we were here, searching and finding at least some bits of the way—and lightning conductors to draw down blessings from on high?"[2]

There are particular "stones" I would like to add to the cairns, as we move into the twenty-first century, which I think are being formed as a result of the AIDS experience. These concepts are not new, but our perception of them and the value system they influence is still vital and in formation. The "stones" are as follows:

- a twentieth-century theology of suffering
- the rediscovery of story, tradition, and symbol
- the challenge of the feminine to the patriarchy
- the healing ministry of the Church

A Twentieth-Century Theology of Suffering

The English theologian Jim Cotter has written:

Some of the quarrying of the stones will come from suffering and the suffering of God. Even if God is sustaining us, we have to bear the burden of the quarrying if we are pioneers. We have to go down into the roughness of the stones and the glaring heat. At the bottom of the quarry, when we thought we were getting somewhere, we have to realize that we cannot of ourselves become perfect—indeed that all our expertise, effort and reputation have to be shattered to fragments.[3]

The failures and successes of any century have never been so carefully recorded as those of the twentieth century. The first half was captured on newsreels; the second half boldly invaded our homes on television. We can see footage of the gas-filled trenches of the First World War; the incredible piles of human remains of the Holocaust; the first nuclear devastation of a people; the carnage of Vietnam; the assassination of our dreamers and prophets; and the horrors of mass hunger on this planet. The challenge to any religious system that will survive into the twenty-first century is to somehow make sense of the suffering recorded on miles of film and videotape. We cannot erase, fast-forward, or even substitute it for a fantasy movie. The images challenge the Church to develop an honest theology of suffering. Again, this means delving into our deepest past and choosing our most powerful symbols.

Not surprisingly, AIDS-phobia in churches has emerged around the use of the common cup, which in both Jewish and

Christian traditions has symbolized bitterness, pain, and suffering. This controversy at a local level can be a great opportunity, not only for AIDS education, but for a reevaluation of the local church's commitment to the suffering. The Christian eucharist is seen as solidarity with Christ in his suffering, sharing in his Passion through death and resurrection. "Christ has died; Christ is risen; Christ will come again!" The twentieth-century Church has largely ignored a vast tradition of "theology of suffering," except for the work of Barth, Moltmann, and Bonhoeffer, who maximized their exposure to the rise of fascism and its fruit, the Holocaust. I was glad to hear a comment by Matthew Fox, the creationist theologian, critical of most contemporary American New Age religion for ignoring the realities of suffering and being an obvious escape from it. In our contemporary hedonism and religious anesthesia we can make Christ resemble whatever we want or need. Fox says, "A cosmic Christ without wounds is not *the* Christ, and those who celebrate a Christ without wounds are false mystics."[4]

Throughout history the "suffering God" has been affirmed. The writings of St. Paul Ignatius of Antioch spoke of the "suffering God." At the Council of Ephesus of C.E. 431, the crucial step toward understanding the identity of Christ's pain with the pain of God was taken in the formula concerning the divine motherhood of Mary. Mary, proclaimed Ephesus, was Theotokos, the "God-bearer," the Mother of God. She was the mother of the flesh of God. This assertion, after centuries of reflection, led to the "Theopaschite" (literally, God-suffering) formula, the claim that God has suffered in the flesh. As Gregory of Nazienzen has stressed, "We needed a God made flesh and put to death in order that we could live again."[5] Gregory spoke of the blood of God and the crucified God, a term later taken up by Luther who speaks of the "deus crucifixus."

In reflecting and brooding on the suffering of God in the Christ event, Christians have been led to see the extension of the Passion into the life of the human family. Karl Barth expressed this well: "So dark is our situation that God himself must enter and occupy it in order that it may be light. We cannot fully understand the Christian 'God with us' without the greatest astonishment at the glory of the Divine Grace and the greatest horror at our own plight."[6]

Jürgen Moltmann's contribution to this theology is more radical than Barth's. In the theme of a suffering God we are actually confronted with a view of God opposed to the God of conventional theism.

> With the Christian message of the cross of Christ, something new and strange has entered the metaphysical world. For this faith must understand the deity of God from the event of the suffering and death of the Son of God, and thus bring about a fundamental change in the orders of being of metaphysical thought. It must think of the suffering of Christ as the power of God and the death of Christ as God's potentiality.[7]

Moltmann's definition of Christian faith sees God as supremely revealed in the suffering of the human Christ; therefore, it has important consequences for our response to the presence of God in the sufferings of others. God bears in God's heart all the wounds of the human family; through our encounter with pain and suffering, we come to see the meaning of God's presence in the world. The cross, symbolic of God's love and commitment to humankind and all Creation, is a rejection of the "apathetic" God who is incapable of suffering.

This passionate involvement of God in the pain of the world brings about a real transformation of men and women. Warner Traynham, rector of St. John's Church, Los Angeles, once noted in an AIDS mass sermon that the most marginalized groups who have suffered persecution by the host community are "God's agents of change" in the world.[8] They have the least invested in the oppressing society and are therefore the most open to the spirit of change and transformation. Jesus' saying, that the poor are always with us, was descriptive rather than prescriptive. A theology of suffering is a practical theology.

Douglas John Hall, in *Lighten Our Darkness: Towards an Indigenous Theology of the Cross,* says, "The theology of the cross can never be a brilliant statement about the brokenness of life: it has to be a broken statement about life's brokenness because it participates in what it seeks to describe."[9]

Monica Furlong, the English writer and theologian, described the strange connection between suffering and spirituality. Those who were most "perceptive" and vibrant in her life were six people who had all suffered in some way through physical, emotional, or societal handicaps.

The people whom I have loved best have all known some experience akin to this. One of them stammered, two experienced severe maternal deprivation, two were homosexual, one was seriously rejected and bullied by his peers. What made them special was not the original wound, but the fact that it seemed to open a door, which in others remained closed, a door which led into a landscape of joy. This does not happen automatically as a result of injury—people can be injured, yet remain unaware—but I know of no one who seems able to talk of this landscape without having known the pain first.[10]

John Fortunato gives us a simple spiritual exercise. Say, "Here is God. Here is God." He challenges us to chant this phrase for a whole day, like saying an Eastern mantra.

Now sometimes the words will come very easily, like—like when you have some pious thought, or it is a lovely day, or something wonderful has happened in the world. Yes, at those sweet moments, the warm fuzzies of religious sentiment will enfold you like so many delightful cirrus clouds.

But now try your mantra when you pass a rat-infested abandoned lot in a slum; or have some murderous, hateful thought; or read about the latest terrorist attack; or hear on the news about the most recent rape in your city or about another natural disaster. Now watch the warm fuzzies turn into cold pricklies.[11]

Fortunato's book *Embracing the Exile* develops this theme further, for gay and lesbian people in particular. His subsequent book, *AIDS: The Spiritual Dilemma,* struggles with some of the larger vocational questions asked by the AIDS-affected community. The great challenge is to somehow believe that in the horror and tragedy of this disease is the very place where God's love and activity are realized. For many of us familiar with "gentle Jesus meek and mild" and "prosperity is your divine right" theological perspectives, AIDS does not fit our comfortable but infantile pegholes. The AIDS experience in the latter part of the twentieth century may be the final tragedy to break the dam of denial that has been so carefully constructed to hold back the pain of this century. Owning, articulating, and healing that pain is another great challenge to the Church.

The Rediscovery of Story, Tradition, and Symbol

The most significant impact by AIDS on the "psyche of America" is the stirring up of primitive images of plague, disease, and death. Judith Ross at the University of California/Los Angeles has written about the language we use around AIDS. A word can be so charged spiritually, politically, and socially that we need to attend to what we say. She describes the media's use of the word *plague,* for example, as conjuring up a religious aura.[12] Many of us first learned about plague in Sunday school: God's punishment on the Egyptians. Twentieth-century mainstream Christianity has virtually abdicated this powerful reservoir of language, words, stories, and symbols to the fundamentalist Christians, who use it for their own political and theological agendas.

Dan Matthews, rector of Trinity Church in Manhattan, sees the correlation between a society that is morally and ethically bankrupt and a society that has forgotten its tradition of storytelling. Within our diverse cultural heritage of stories and traditions, is a sense of solidarity with one's identity, community, and the past. These stories give shape and meaning to our existence; they teach ethical and moral values and help to bring comfort and solace in times of adversity and hardship.[13]

One of the delights of returning to my Irish roots is to listen wistfully to my family (usually after a few drinks!) as they tell their stories about one another: dead brothers and sisters, neighbors and friends. Usually, amongst the laughter and tears, exaggeration and expletives, there is truth and integrity; the narratives reveal the meaning of their lives. Their stories *had* to be told.

Matthew's ideas challenge the mainstream churches to get back to "biblical Christianity." That we Anglicans wince at this term proves the point that we have allowed the extremists to claim our wellspring. "Without the vision, the people will perish." Many of us have escaped from so-called Bible-centered churches scarred, emotionally and spiritually, by past experiences; we may not want to open those old wounds. However, during the AIDS crisis we may survive and emerge with greater spiritual maturity only if we are grounded in the stories of the mighty acts of God in the lives of people such as ourselves.

The Jesus story has recently been brought to public attention by the film *The Last Temptation of Christ.* The controversy even placed Jesus' face on the front of *Time* magazine, illustrating the contemporary interest and confusion about the Jesus story. The Jesus story is our most powerful symbol of victory over a seemingly pointless, premature, and cruel death. Many of us have been renewed in our faith by the power of this particular story through our AIDS ministries.

One of the most moving pieces of writing to come out of the AIDS experience was by Richard Smith, of St. Augustine's parish in Santa Monica, who died last year. He overlayed the stations of the cross on Jesus' journey to Golgotha with the final journey of a person with AIDS. Not only was this a helpful spiritual exercise for Smith, but it was also an effective way of communicating to deeply religious people who *know* that story; they have experienced AIDS in their own lives and faced their own mortality.[14]

Dan Matthews describes the need for communities of faith to tell not only the traditional biblical stories but also their *own* stories; this is a great challenge to those coming out of the AIDS experience. How do individuals and groups who have been denied their past and traditions tell "the whole story"? Earlier this century, in Wales, those children who spoke only Welsh were humiliated by their Anglo teachers and classmates and forced to deny their roots and traditions. American society has many individuals and groups who have been forced to forget their stories, either through choice, shame, or socioeconomic pressures. Blacks, Hispanics, Native Americans, working-class immigrants, women, gay men, and lesbians all have been denied opportunities to hear and learn their own stories. Or, what they have been told is so sentimentalized that it anesthetizes, rather than empowers. Dare we begin to tell the story of the Christian Church and its impact on this list of disinherited communities?

In Pasadena today our church stands for social and racial justice. However, forty years ago we had our share of anti-Semites who wanted to keep Jews out of Pasadena and white supremacists who wanted to keep blacks in their place. Telling the whole story will not be easy for any of us. Rediscovering those words and traditions and creating those communities who can tell, listen, and pass on the stories, developed out of their own experience, is a challenge to the church. It will be from this foundation that our value system will be reformed and renewed.

Our collective words in the AIDS experience have been hard to find. The ambitious "theologizing of AIDS" may occupy most of our lives in the attempt to "make sense" of it all. Two "cultic" experiences are worth noting here because they describe how important tradition is for us. Cotter says, "The cairn needs to be reshaped as it meets your particular and living experience and environment. You may use much the same stones, but the cairn needs to be rebuilt. It may be some of us are not yet cairn-builders: all we are ready to do is to take a stone from a particular cairn and reshape it through the uniqueness of our own experi-ence—we will have to spend time working as craftsmen and women at work, with the aim of learning what s/he does rather than trying to copy his style and merely imitate or repeat a de-sign."[15] Like "collective mantras," the cultic experiences of AIDS have reaffirmed a deep sense of spirituality in communities tradi-tionally rejected by organized religion or themselves suspicious of things spiritual and cultic.

The Names Project quilt, or the National AIDS Quilt, which has traveled to every major city in the United States in the past twelve months, does more than anything else I have experienced to express the gravity, horror, and the diversity of people and talent lost in the AIDS crisis. What gentle loving is expressed in those handcrafted panels! It was displayed in Detroit (a provi-dential coincidence!) at the same time and in the same location as the 69th General Convention of the Episcopal Church in July 1988.

The National Episcopal AIDS Coalition (NEAC) spent several months planning its participation at General Convention and its advocacy of nine AIDS-related resolutions, which were adopted. The campaign was highly orchestrated, politically sophisticated, and successful overall. However, we were not prepared, as a Convention or as NEAC, for the Wednesday morning AIDS Heal-ing Service and dedication of the Episcopal AIDS memorial quilt panels led by our presiding bishop, Edmond Browning. We sol-emnly walked downstairs through a corridor lined with three-by-six-foot panels of the quilt, inscribed with the names of four thousand people who have died as a result of AIDS. Many of us, liturgical leaders usually composed at memorials, succumbed to tears as we mourned our friends, lovers, and parishioners. In the next few days, many convention delegates, having had little pre-vious exposure to the AIDS crisis, were visibly moved by their visit to the quilt in the exposition hall. I interpret this as a sign of true compassion from people who may not fully understand the complexities of AIDS. This is a sign of hope for a church that may be confused and fearful about all sorts of issues but can weep openly as it embraces the pain of this latter-day holocaust.

The second cultic experience, rooted much more in the liturgical tradition of the Episcopal Church, was a series of AIDS masses held in the Los Angeles diocese from 1985 through 1987. The first occurred upon my return from London and the bedside of Frank, one of my closest friends, who died as a result of AIDS. In my overwhelming grief, painful loss, and unfocused anger, I had nowhere to go for relief. I was dismayed upon arriving at my home parish that Sunday morning to discover that a mariachi band would perform at the eucharist; I endured an experience spiritually irrelevant to my immediate crisis. Later that day I attended the first AIDS mass, at St. Augustine's parish in Santa Monica. The spacious building was full of gay men: weeping, angry, many unchurched, all frightened. Somehow the familiar words, readings, prayers, and liturgical settings filled me with the Spirit, and I found comfort and meaning in it all, although I still cannot articulate what I felt. I know only that it was important to find a place to go where others knew what I was feeling and where we could grieve and hope together.

This is not an alien ministry for the Church. We have been doing this sort of thing for years; it is the *least* we can do in a crisis we still do not fully comprehend. Frank's death marked my own initiation into AIDS ministry, and I had the privilege of coordinating the next seven AIDS masses throughout the diocese, with the assistance of our suffragan bishop, Oliver B. Garver, Jr. The same hungry, tear-filled look in the eyes of the congregations tied each of the events together. Our church's ministry, mission, and message through those masses lived in ways the majority of our Sunday congregations could not comprehend. The AIDS masses, more than anything else in the past five years in our diocese, have shown the local gay community our seriousness in welcoming them into parish communities and our intention to create a more compassionate and diverse church. They have lost many friends, lovers, family members, and they now fear for their own future. Public health authorities tell us that 30 to 50 percent of urban gay males may have already been exposed to the human immunodeficiency virus; a spiritual program and supportive parish community is the anchor many need in the storm of AIDS.

From time to time I remind my heterosexual colleagues at All Saints Church that every time gay or lesbian people sit in our pews, they return to the place they first heard that their person and/or their love was not good. This was often tragically "acted out" by some congregations or priests through overt acts of expulsion or excommunication. In the storm of AIDS, people move either into denial or deeper into a spiritual program. Some parishes actually have something to offer. Those gay and lesbian parishioners are in church to do some very difficult spiritual integration within themselves and within the family of faith.

I predict the total integration of gay and lesbian people within mainstream Christianity within the next twenty years. The decision to integrate lies not so much with the heterosexual membership of the Church but with those gays and lesbians who seek to deepen their faith and to reclaim their place among the People of God. They will have the ability and courage to tell their stories to their heterosexual brothers and sisters, witnessing to the presence of God in their lives. As Episcopalians, we may be one of the first prophetic communities in the United States where this will happen.

The Challenge of the Feminine to the Patriarchy

Barbara Walker's book *The Crone* begins with the premise that the basis for man's sexism is his fear of death.[16] Women, as demonstrated in religious stories such as the Creation Fall, were seen as "death bringers" and reminders of human mortality. Walker's book traces the historic oppression of women in the last three to five thousand years, particularly by the Judeo-Christian patriarchy. Her evidence and theory are compelling. The prepatriarchal deity was feminine: a trinity of Virgin, Mother, and Destroyer. Time was cyclical, not linear; the Mother Goddess destroyed in order to recreate and resurrect, like the Indian goddess Vishnu. The Christian God was a father, a manufacturer who could not give birth but created. Some aspects of feminine religion were maintained by the patriarchy, but many of its powerful symbols were feared.

How frightening AIDS seems in our sexist culture! The root of homophobia is sexism. Our anger at the homosexual male is partly because he does not act like a "real man" but behaves "as a woman." This simplistic rationale is important to understanding the spiritual and cultural enormity we are dealing with as we involve ourselves in the AIDS experience. We are not only flagrantly talking about the taboo subjects of death to an already terrified sexist culture, but we are also talking about the taboo subject of homosexuality: a double whammy! It appears our unenviable vocation is to somehow force our society to confront death and our own mortality. The scientific/medical/mortuarial "industrial complex" has us all (nearly) convinced that death is no problem for our generation. Fortunato says,

> Most everyone would agree that it could not have come at a worse time. Here we had almost succeeded in obliterating death from our consciousness. We had worked so hard for so long. More than a century of progressively hiding the Grim Reaper, or euphemising death, of phoneying up corpses, of putting fake grass around the hole and leaving before the box was lowered. And we were within a hair's breadth of our goal.[17]

Fortunato sees the embracing of sensuality as an important feminine and Christian action:

> God given and wonderful, part of our experience of life is inevitably running headlong into death. To live fully in one's body is to experience sooner or later this body will rot—whether it is taut and muscled or fat and flabby—it will rot.[18]

Fortunato also links death's representation by women to include gay men. He goes on to say,

> There is a sense in which gay people have always represented mortality to the world—non-procreational sexuality, 'a non-birth experience' which as experienced at some primordial level is the same as death.[19]

Here we connect with the role of the feminine in the AIDS experience, particularly the role of women and gay men.

Last year I was invited to speak on AIDS at an in-service training for members of the leading Roman Catholic hospital system in California. The evening before the conference I had dinner with the faculty, the president of the corporation and her staff, and some leading hospital administrators. They shared stories of their work situations, and I saw that, at the core level, they were profoundly sexist: male physicians, politicians, and insurance bureaucrats over against some very powerful women in health

care. Something clicked inside my head. Mother Church, or
rather *Father Church,* has too much invested in the existing
patriarchy to want change. The AIDS issue, still a "hot potato" in
the Church, is but an outward manifestation of deeper and more
serious problems.

At a profound, dark, unconscious level the feminine, whether
a woman, a woman priest, a gay man, or the Deity, frightens and
disturbs us in a way we do not yet fully understand. Yet without
the feminine there is no birth—no life—no authentic spirituality,
mysticism, or healing. Many of Christianity's most important
"feminine" symbols—the holy city, vessels, the tree of life, the
earth, the cave, the mountain, and the fort—must not be obscured. Erich Neumann said, "Whenever we encounter a symbol
of rebirth, we have to do it with a matriarchal transformation
mystery, and this is true even when its symbolism or interpretation bears a patriarchal guise."[20] "Father religions," wrote Eric
Erikson, "have mother Churches."[21]

Kenneth Leech's book *Experiencing God* has a helpful chapter
entitled "God the Mother."[22] He notes that the twelfth century
was a crucial period for the reemergence of feminine symbols of
the divine, ironically, used by men. We also see a feminization of
language in that era as well as a deepening interiority of devotion
and mysticism. Our own era has gone through similar changes in
perception and language.

The twelfth century was the period of the Beguines, the first
women's movement in Western history. This was also a period in
which the humanity of Christ came to be emphasized as part of
a general shift in spirituality from atonement-resurrection-law-
judgment motifs toward an increased stress on Creation and Incarnation. This shift of emphasis, the influence of women, is
very important. Women created and developed devotion to the
infant Jesus and to the sacred heart and wounds. Women mystics
were responsible for the introduction of the Feast of Corpus
Christi. In the same century, we see the first flowering of Jesus as
"Mother." These shifts are found in the writings of such notables
as Hildegard of Bingen, Aelred of Rievaulx, and Anselm of
Canterbury. Out of this rich tradition from the patristic to the
medieval period, Dame Julian of Norwich in the fourteenth century created a whole cycle of divine maternal activity.[23]

Not until the eighteenth century was the feminine dimension
of God reemphasized by a variety of fringe Protestant groups,

notably the Shakers. In the Shaker view, male redemption was necessarily incomplete, so they looked for a future female redeemer in the figure of Ann Lee. Central to Shaker theology was the view that there must be a second manifestation of the Christ, this time in female form; this rediscovery of the feminine dimension in God has rightly been seen as "the most significant Shaker contribution to American religion."[24]

The Shakers thought of God in four persons: Father, Mother (Wisdom), Son, and Daughter. Similar ideas appeared in the Mormon movement and Christian Science. So while conventional mainstream Christianity proclaimed a masculine God, the fringe heretical movements restated the feminine dimension of God previously found within orthodox Christian tradition.

In our day the work of Carl Jung has shed new light on discovering the feminine in God, with special emphasis on Mary. For Jung, the doctrine of the assumption of Mary pointed to a great recovery in theology. He wrote:

The Assumptio Mariae paves the way not only for the divinity of Theotokos (i.e., her ultimate recognition as a goddess) but also the quaternity. At the same time, matter is included in the metaphysical realm together with the corrupting principle of the cosmos, evil.[25]

This development from Trinity to Quaternity is a natural progression for Jung and has profound implications for churches already struggling with more inclusive language. Orthodox church leaders, including the present pope, are moving toward a strong Marian theology while maintaining antifeminist positions.

From Mary, who in her Magnificat proclaims that salvation has to do with justice, there flowers authentic commitment to the rest of humanity, our brothers and sisters, especially for the poorest and the most needy, and to the transformation of society.[26]

Rosemary Ruether comments on a more radical Marian theology and links it to the theology of liberation:

The church is the ongoing Christ as the liberated poor who continue to serve and liberate others. And also those who suffer, as those who pay the price for their struggle for liberation. Mary, as the personified Church. The liberated poor cannot become models for continued subjugation, but rather of messianic empowerment. She is 'alter Christus.' She is the messianic people who continues the liberating action of God in the world. The last becomes first, and the first last, a poor women of despised race is the head of the Church.[27]

When historians look back from the twenty-first century to our crumbling patriarchal society, with its principal *raison d'être* the maintenance of a patriarchal Christian church, they will trace the beginnings of the transformation to the early 1960s during the pontificate of John XXIII. It is ironic that this unlikely symbol of the patriarchy, while saying his prayers on a feast day of Mary, should conceive the idea for a renewed church. His papacy marked the end of an era, and the church, catholic and reformed, is still reeling from that radical intervention.

Sexuality and the feminine are still the major issues in our branch of the Church, whether during the heated debates on homosexuality at the recent General Convention or in the Anglican bishops agreeing on the ordination of women, the consecration of women bishops, and the permitting of polygamy in some Anglican provinces.

The AIDS experience heightens and makes more immediate these important areas of conflict and controversy. Time for talking and theologizing is limited in the midst of so much fear, suffering, and ignorance. Many of the patriarchal concepts and value systems currently being challenged have a vested interest in ignoring or containing theological exploration into the areas of sexuality, homosexuality, the feminine, and death. This puts us in a difficult place. As Cotter describes it:

> In a time when there is no overriding religious interpretation of life, this spiritual way will struggle with the language and meaning of faith. Its practitioners will feel uneasy with the institutions of religion, however loyal they may be: filial disobedience might be the phrase. In some ways they will be on the edge, not totally committed to the present, listening for a word to come, alert to an emerging future that may carry forward the life and purposes of faith to better effect.[28]

The Healing Ministry of the Church

The stories of Jesus healing the ill comprise the most memorable aspects of the ministry of Jesus. Our knowledge and experience through the intervening two millenia have moved us into another, very different, world, a world of technological and scientific progress inspired by people who were also healers. Many people of faith, some inspired by the memories of Jesus, created whole institutions devoted to healing and maintaining health. Cotter calls this "a supportive and critical solidarity" with some segment of the secular world. He sees this as an important expression of faith for some, as much as prayer or worship.[29] This spiritual way is the opposite of "soul culture" for it embraces the partial, the messy, and the embodied. Inevitably this way tackles the sexual and the political, the fleshly body and the body politic. Supportive and critical solidarity involves a celebration of what goes right, a repenting of what goes wrong, the receiving of forgiveness, and a search for words of meaning in this particular endeavor. For many of us, AIDS has provided the impetus for a "supportive and critical solidarity" with other healers, particularly in the health care industry.

Our involvement and response to persons with AIDS, their caregivers, and their families have compelled many of us to look at the relationship between human health, the ministry and teaching of Jesus, and the multi-billion-dollar industry we call "health care." I used to wonder why sixteenth-century Europeans were so gullible as to buy indulgences from the pope to enable the construction of St. Peter's basilica. Our grandchildren will look back in history and wonder why we so gullibly allowed the insurance and medical industries to dictate the quality and availability of health care, while at the same time we tolerated environmental pollution, carcinogenic pesticides, food preservatives, high levels of tobacco and alcohol consumption—evils that will have had such an impact on the health of people at the beginning of the twenty-first century.

A Retrospective Flashback

What might this era look like in twenty years? Imagine living in a new century where health care is very different; look back at the influence of AIDS-related care on the new system, as well as the role of the Church in health and healing.

The AIDS epidemic was the final straw that ended the cycle of death caused by poor disease prevention and health maintenance. When the insurance and medical industries realized it was more cost-effective to educate and prevent the spread of AIDS among the general population, other prevention lobbies—lung cancer, chemical abuse, and heart disease, among them—began to gain ground. Disease prevention has never been a *cause célèbre* in American health care, but the system became so overutilized—people with lung cancer, heart disease, seventy-thousand people with AIDS—that something had to give.

As costs soared, the health care marketplace became frantic. Many hospitals closed, unable to survive in the highly competitive marketplace. Medicine became more and more technological, requiring multi-million-dollar scanners, highly skilled surgical specialists, and other such highly priced equipment and personnel. It became the practice to get the patient out of the hospital into home-based nursing or attendant care. The people with AIDS were the first significant patient population to be so managed. Not only did they cause "public relations" problems for most hospitals, but the levels of care needed could not justify the thousand-dollar-per-day cost to keep them there.

Case management, a community-based discharge planning and health management system developed originally for seniors, seemed most appropriate for the growing AIDS population. Many of them were cared for at home or in specialized day-care centers, and these also became more popular with seniors. Many nursing homes were full, understaffed, and poorly managed; they became like human warehouses, resulting in a shift in practices. Community leaders became more involved with the terminally ill and incapacitated. People from churches, hospices, and hospitals became active in the ethical, economic, and programmatic development of catastrophic and terminal care with these populations.

In the early 1980s, smaller community-based hospices sprang up all over the country, some started by churches and other community groups to take care of AIDS patients. Some were illegal and could not be licensed as either residential or health care facilities. A new category of smaller community-based hospices was created, which then developed their own hospice protocols and provided physician training in the care of the terminally ill.

The highly technological and economically centered medical and insurance complexes were finally challenged by a series of religious, bioethical, and humanitarian fronts. In 1988, sixty million Americans were excluded from proper health insurance and medical care because of their employment situations. Emergency and indigent programs all over the country were closed due to lack of funds. Health care became the leading issue of the 1992 presidential campaign; the electorate provided a mandate for universal health care in every state by the end of the twentieth century. The reforms of Willis Bowen, secretary of the Department of Health and Human Services in 1987, provided medical coverage for catastrophic disease for seniors. Senator Edward Kennedy, the Reverend Jesse Jackson, and Surgeon-General C. Everett Koop helped to shape a new national health care strategy. The AIDS epidemic was the final straw causing the collapse of one of the most wasteful and inefficient health services in the world.

The AIDS epidemic also influenced two other major health-related fields that became more integrated: psychology and immunology. Research at UCLA and other schools in the late 1980s described important links between the body's immune function, stress, psychological ill health, and the oppression of various ethnic and minority groups, as well as the importance of spiritual programs dealing with self-image; self-esteem; participating in small, intimate community experiences; human touch; and healthy relationships. In the 1990s, interest grew in the relationship between compulsive behavior and disease, particularly related to chemical use, sexual compulsivity, and overeating. Many variations of the twelve-step Alcoholics Anonymous program were adapted to these populations. All these programs were assisted by a strong religious presence that provided seed monies for programs, leadership development, and facilities.

At the same time, traditional healing services and New Age techniques of imaging, meditation, massage, touch therapy, and support groups often became a regular part of parish programs. These helped people deal with family and work-related stress, loss, lack of community amid the growing popularity of non-theistic New Age communities. As a result of these influences, the traditional churches further developed their programs of initiation, storytelling, Christian education, and liturgies, placing special emphasis on eucharistic celebrations that included healing services with the laying-on-of-hands and annointing with oil. Many of these programs were tried experimentally with AIDS-affected populations (some of whom became church members) and leadership within the clergy and laity. These early ministries also influenced the recruitment, training, and support of lay leadership in the Church. The early AIDS movement was basically a lay volunteer movement.

A major synthesis of mental health and physical health was established in California in 1984, growing out of the anonymous testing programs for HIV antibodies. The state-funded program linked the blood tests with pre- and post-test counseling. Many of the local community organizations refused to sign contracts to begin the testing unless adequate mental health support was included. The Genetically Handicapped Person's Program had established the principle of the co-dependancy of mental health and physical health for people who were genetically disabled, but the AIDS crisis pushed this principle into other areas. More than any disease, AIDS forced the professional health care provider to move beyond his or her expertise and to work as part of a community team. The religious community did much to give "glue" to this synergy, encouraging people to develop more than one expertise. This is reflected in the skills of many of the people in leadership positions in the AIDS-affected community.

Steps to Get There

All the events and programs covered in this essay are occurring at some level within religious and health-related communities of our nation. The seeds of the new community and new health care are already sown and germinating around and within us. To encourage these developments, we need to foster discussion that may evolve into the establishment of prevention and care programs at parish and institutional levels (seminaries, hospitals, schools, and dioceses) where these issues are engaged.

Our church must continue its commitment to fight institutional sexism at every level of church participation for women to ensure a healthy community. The first moves to ordain women began more than twenty years ago; it has taken that long to make it possible for women to exercise full leadership in our church. The same commitment and energy needs to be exercised fighting homophobia and racism within and outside the church. Homophobia is the largest single factor in the lack of early AIDS prevention and care programs throughout the United States; 63 percent of persons with AIDS in this country are homosexual. The church can address this successfully by developing congregational resources on homosexuality, within the spectrum of human sexuality, as well as by further developing pastoral programs to include gay and lesbian people in the life of the church and to assure access to ordination for anyone regardless of sexual orientation. If the past six years are any gauge of the future, we also will have to monitor political and legislative attempts to isolate persons with AIDS, or those suspected as having AIDS, from the general population. The church has an important role in guarding basic civil rights, particularly the rights of minority populations.

With the formation of the National Episcopal AIDS Coalition, we have a vehicle for communication among the existing AIDS ministries in the country. This will enable the experiences and model programs now existing in parishes and institutions to be shared with groups not yet active in AIDS ministry.

The AIDS crisis requires us to be highly sensitive to cultural values. One of our greatest challenges at the local level will be to take programs proven successful in the Anglo community and adapt them to the cultural perspectives of the black and Hispanic communities. We also will need to create new ethnically sensitive programs of care and prevention, and we must continue to underpin professional response to the crisis with trained and supported volunteers. The church is in a unique position with minority communities to develop leadership networking and community organizing around AIDS prevention and services.

Theologians, educators, pastors, and persons with AIDS must continue to "theologize" and reflect on their experiences in the midst of the crisis. This work represents an important cairn in our understanding of the AIDS epidemic to this point, showing our commitment to be a compassionate church as we seek the will of God on these issues.

References

1. M. Furlong, *Traveling In* (London: Hodder, 1971), p. 25.
2. B. Urquhard, cited in Jim Cotter, *The Cairns Network* (Exeter, England: Cairns Publications, 1987).
3. Cotter, *Cairns Network,* p. 4.
4. M. Fox, "Christian Mysticism and Peace" (Lecture, Pasadena, Calif., May 1987); from the author's personal notes.
5. J. Meyendorff, *Christ in Eastern Christian Thought* (New York: St. Vladimirs Press, 1975). pp. 69–89.
6. K. Barth, *Church Dogmatics,* vol. 4, pt. 1, cited in Kenneth

Leech, *Experiencing God* (San Francisco: Harper & Row, 1985), p. 302.

7. J. Moltmann, *The Crucified God* (London: SCM Press, 1974), pp. 214–15.

8. Sermon delivered at an AIDS Mass, Long Beach, Calif., March 1987; from the author's personal notes.

9. D.J. Hall, *Lighten Our Darkness: Towards an Indigenous Theology of the Cross* (Philadelphia: Westminster Press, 1976), p. 117.

10. Furlong, *Traveling In,* p. 28.

11. J. Fortunato, *AIDS: The Spiritual Dilemma* (San Francisco: Harper & Row, 1987), p. 100.

12. J. Ross, "The Language of AIDS" (Lecture, March 1987); from the author's personal notes.

13. D. Matthews (Lecture delivered to the Vestry of All Saints Church, Pasadena, Calif., at a retreat in May 1987); from the author's personal notes.

14. R. Smith, *Stations* (Privately printed by Holy Nativity Parish, Westchester, Calif., 1987).

15. Cotter, *Cairns Network.* p. 4.

16. B. Walker, *The Crone* (San Francisco: Harper & Row, 1985).

17. Fortunato, *AIDS,* p. 69.

18. Ibid., p. 80.

19. Ibid.

20. E. Neumann, *The Great Mother: An Analysis of the Archetype* (New York: Pantheon Books, 1955), p. 59.

21. E. Erikson, *Young Man Luther: A Study in Psychoanalysis and History* (New York: W.W. Norton, 1958), p. 263.

22. Leech, *Experiencing God.*

23. See M. Reeves, *The Influence of Prophecy in the Middle Ages* (Oxford: Clarendon Press, 1969). Also see C.W. Bynum, *Jesus as Mother: Studies in the Spirituality of the Middle Ages* (Berkeley: University of California Press, 1982), p. 14.

24. S.M. Setta, *From Ann the Christ to Holy Mother Wisdom* (Fall Equinox Press, 1980).

25. C.G. Jung, cited in Leech, *Experiencing God,* p. 369.

26. Pope John Paul II, address to the Puebla conference of Latin American bishops, cited by Rosemary Radford Ruether in *The Witness* 62(October 1979): p. 15.

27. Ruether, op. cit.; also *Sexism and God Talk* (Boston: Beacon Press, 1983), p. 152.

28. Cotter, *Cairns Network,* p. 6.
29. Ibid. p. 5.

Biographical Note

Albert J. Ogle is a priest of the Anglican Church of Ireland. His divinity degree was awarded with honors by University College of North Wales. He did further theological study at Trinity College, Dublin, and additional studies at the University of London Institute of Education and the University of Ireland at Maynooth. He has served parishes in Belfast and Dublin, directed an inner city project in London, and was licensed to officiate in the Diocese of Los Angeles in 1982. He has held staff positions at the Gay and Lesbian Community Services Center in Hollywood, was founder of the Triangle Project for high-risk youth, was director of planning and development at the AIDS Project Los Angeles, and initiated and developed the AIDS Interfaith Council of Southern California. He was coauthor of the "Meyers Plan," published by the Health Policy and Research Foundation of California, a statewide needs assessment and plan for AIDS treatment services in California for 1987–91. He was a consultant with the Episcopal Commission on AIDS Ministry for the Diocese of Los Angeles and, since November 1987, has been executive director of the All Saints AIDS Service Center in Pasadena.

Scraps from an Organic Quilt
Ruth Black

But this is not the story of a life
It is the story of lives, knit together,
overlapping in succession, rising
again from grave after grave.[1]

Introduction: Transformation of a Metaphor

Martin Marty, in the foreword to John Booty's *The Episcopal Church in Crisis,* posed this problem:

> It is one thing to tell the story of the remote past, after most documents have been lost, after almost all have been picked over. It is another matter to sort out details from a documentary blizzard—there have not yet been enough burned libraries, destroyed attics—and find the significance in stories about people still alive or about people we remember.[2]

Whether we address history or theology in the AIDS pandemic, those of us in the trenches have difficulty with perspective. Events, people, feelings, memories are raw for us. Pervading whatever we say or write is the most recent feeling or the sense of grief or anger. At least, in my own case this is true.

Thus, I commend Albert Ogle for tackling the difficulties of sorting through the "documentary blizzard"! I commend him also for the image of cairns and the four areas of transformation he sees now and in the future. I will focus on these indirectly rather than head-on.

Futuristic projection is never easy and is made more difficult now because of our own lack of distance from the experience. Some of us have participated in so many "AIDS Updates" and workshops that, like Ned in "The Normal Heart," we confess, "Felix, I am so sick of statistics, and numbers, and body counts and how-manys . . . and everyday . . . there are only more numbers. . . ."[3] This morning's paper bore the headline, "Study says AIDS spreading worldwide at one victim per minute." At that rate, from the time of the beginning of our symposium until its end, 2,640 new people will be infected with the human immunodeficiency virus. That fact is stunning.

On first reading Albert Ogle's "Transformation," however, I was overwhelmed by another sort of documentary blizzard: rich detail drawn from many sources. As I began to outline my own response, I found it difficult and searched rather for a metaphor. The image of cairns, of stone markers along the way, dropped into my stream of consciousness. Ripples diverged. The more I struggled with a linear response to the essay, the more none came that had life for me. Only circles, ever-widening ripples remained: of story, image, symbol, connection. Biblical rocks surfaced: the stone for a pillar for Jacob at Beth-El and my own story in a hospital room; the smooth stone secured in David's sling to slay Goliath (1 Sam. 17:40ff.) and the metaphor of AIDS felling the giant health care system; the confession of Peter and the "Rock" on which I stand in my own chaplaincy; the woman at Jacob's (stone) well leaving the pitcher (her traditional task) to tell her story; the stones *not* thrown at the woman taken in adultery and the protective stone wall of legislation built by some of the AIDS resolutions at General Convention.

On first reading I longed for another cairn: the stone rolled away from an empty tomb. The calendar seemed fixed on Holy Saturday: the crucifixion done, the waiting for an Easter only dimly viewed, the page yet unturned. I pictured other stones for building, enclosing, supporting: a sloped well of all our stories, memories, hopes (the "wellspring" of which Ogle speaks); stone bridges extended, crossed (the networking of the National Episcopal AIDS Coalition [NEAC]); AIDS homes built, opened, staffed.

The stones softened to flesh (like biblical hearts), then to cloth. "Transformations" became an AIDS Quilt panel connecting the themes of myth, suffering, the feminine, and healing. It seemed to beg scraps from my own supply. In one ludicrous moment I pictured all the presenters/responders patching together our separate panels and the gathering of the one hundred at Church Divinity School of the Pacific in a circle, connecting our pieces into a whole cloth we cannot yet see, the Easter page on the calendar not yet turned.

My response, then, is scrapped and pieced, sometimes by double stitching upon a theme of Ogle's, sometimes by new scraps, sometimes by the overlay of my own at places where my perspective differs from his, sometimes new panels altogether (my stories). A friend advised me, "Ruth, don't try to write feminist theology in response. You already do feminist theology in your life with patients," he said. "Just tell your stories." So I will.

Double Stitching, New Scraps, Overlay, and Panel

A theology of the cross, the Theopaschite formula, informs my own work with terminally ill patients, whether in oncology, on dialysis, or with AIDS. "God as sufferer, God as patient" has become a theology of necessity as well as a practical theology. To those writers mentioned by Ogle, I offer others whose lives in Third World countries place them in marginalized positions. The first is a reminder from the late Bishop Festo Kivingere of Uganda that Christianity is the only faith where God is eternally open, with arms outstretched on the cross, the only faith where there is the "bleeding God who alone can heal bleeding hearts."[4] He notes further that a naked, bleeding God calls people into a totally new community from that of a triumphant, omnipotent God.

Second is Bishop Desmond Tutu's promise of the inevitability of suffering: ". . . a church that does not suffer, cannot be the Church of Jesus Christ. I do not mean we should be masochists. Suffering will seek us out. It is a part of the divine economy of salvation."[5]

Third, Mother Theresa, tending the dying in Calcutta, prays daily for incarnational vision in her "Daily Prayer for the Children's Home": "Dearest Lord, may I see you today and every day in the person of your sick, and whilst nursing them, minister unto you."[6]

John Fortunato's mantra, "Here is God. Here is God. Here is God," further deepens the mystery of suffering for me and also that of the Incarnation.[7]

The following story, patched from much earlier work with a person with AIDS, is my "Jacob" cairn, similar to Ogle's marker after his friend Frank died. Someone asked me how a white, "mainstream," heterosexual woman could possibly minister to PWAs, many of whom are black, some gay, and some intravenous drug abusers. I casually remarked that most often they also ministered to me. But for a while I learned to love the question (to use Rilke's phrase) rather than find an answer. An incarnational answer came in the middle of the night with a healing of my own irrational disease of fear.

It was the middle of the night. I was on call and was summoned by telephone to be with an AIDS patient I did not know. (I think now the ring of the telephone must have sounded to me the way the leper's bell sounded to St. Francis.) All I knew was that his disease had apparently also extended to his central nervous system. He was "hallucinating," the nurse said. "He has had some vision of Jesus and is almost uncontrollable. The security guards won't even go in for fear he'll bite them."

I was afraid. I confess it. I was afraid—an irrational sort of fear. Sometimes I'm afraid I won't know what to do or say with patients in the middle of the night. Sometimes I'm afraid of a large, grieving family, loudly out of control in the hall. Those are nameable, rational fears. This fear was different. It was irrational. I know now it had to do with my own fear of AIDS and, underneath that, my own fear of dying. My own ignorance. My own sense of inadequacy. I was more concerned about myself than I was about my patient as I entered the room.

I remember washing my hands (knowing his susceptibility to any infections I might have) and looking around the room as I entered. Two family members were sitting, almost flattened, against the wall, far from the bed. (Others had abandoned him.) There was a sense of isolation, of estrangement there—not just my own fear, but I think the fear of others in the room. I went to the bed, sat beside him, and asked what I might do to be helpful to him. He wanted to talk to me about his "vision" of Jesus. And he wanted me to pray with him.

As he talked I began to have the warmest sensation of God's presence with me. My fear began to leave. I could hear his own fears: of death, of isolation, of separation. He was no longer an "AIDS patient," a label, but a child of God who happened to have AIDS. Then he asked me to pray with him. "Most of all, please pray that God won't leave me," he said.

I was aware that I had not touched him or even the bed (unusual for me; I usually at least shake hands). It was as if I were holding onto myself and my own fear, arms folded. He folded his hands in a posture of prayer, the way we learned to as children, and asked that I place my hands on top of his as we prayed. It was an unusual request, the first I'd had like that. People often ask me to hold their hand or they reach for mine, but this was different. It was almost as if he wanted someone to enclose his hands as God encloses us always in love. I had the feeling no one had touched him in a long time—that is, for no reason. I did. And I prayed.

I don't remember what I said. It was one of those prayers that I think God prayed through me, or in spite of me. When I opened my eyes, it was as if I had seen this man for the first time: a beautiful child of God. Yes, I think it is fair to say that I saw the face of Christ on this man. I found myself tearful, as if I myself were being healed, rather than he. As I left the room, the words kept coming to me: "I know that my Redeemer lives . . ." and "I was sick and you visited me . . . inasmuch as you have done it to the least of these. . . ."

I saw him only once more after that night. My own fear was gone; my concern was for him. It was as if Jesus had come to me through the man, as if the Holy Spirit had somehow caused both our spirits to begin to overcome our fears: his fear of dying, my own fear of AIDS and beneath it my own of dying. He said he knew God was with him and wouldn't leave him.

It was Sunday. Resurrection Day. It was also the day I felt the white taste of God, formerly stale, turn to flesh on that hospital floor and in my life. As different as he and I were from each other, this patient and I connected at the place of God, a sort of Beth-El. I have a memory of my own fear that allows me to listen more patiently as health care personnel talk away theirs.

Were I to symbolize this cairn in my own life with a panel for the AIDS Quilt, it would consist of a bright background with a large pair of black hands centered as if in prayer. Those would be covered by a much smaller pair of white hands. The cross would be there, the empty tomb, and somewhere a well and a pitcher abandoned in the haste to run and tell the news that I had seen Jesus. The words would read, "The Lord was in this place, and I didn't know it." And Jacob's stone for a pillow would rest nearby.

New permissions for telling our stories within the faith community come from the "stages" movement in theology, medicine, psychology, sociology, regardless of the drawbacks to "stage theory." Kubler-Ross's giving ear to dying patients provides a role model for listening beyond the denial. Piaget, Erikson, Kohlberg, and Gilligan further encourage narrative collecting. James Fowler's theory of stages in spiritual development sees such development as moving from an ego/ethnocentric place to a more theocentric one.[8] Maybe a rereading of his stages will help us, disparate groups, understand how to listen better to each other as we share.

Collections of feminist writings such as Ruether's *Womanguides*,[9] or of the impact of AIDS in stories told in *The Quilt*,[10] or Lon Nungesser's *Epidemic of Courage*[11] help authenticate stories of marginalized people. Recently, the Reverend Nan Arrington Peete chose to tell her story at the Lambeth Conference, rather than instruct by heavier theology.[12] Some of the stories are broken ones; some simply show the "broken myth" or "crushed idol." Many replace old myth with new; others infuse old symbols with new meanings.

I find in story and symbol the challenge of the feminine to the patriarchy. Throughout the AIDS crisis, many men were called to compassionate care and nurture, qualities often called "feminine" by our culture whether applied to God or to human beings. Men who never thought they would be challenged to tasks like changing diapers or fixing food have done these traditionally feminine things as they have tended their brothers with AIDS. Establishing alternative health care facilities, from hospice to home—enclosures rather than skyscrapers—have further moved to the kinds of "hands on" care often associated with roles of females in our culture (mothers, wives, daughters, sisters, nurses, social workers).

The AIDS Quilt, so powerful a symbol of death and resurrection, is a feminine symbol. Barbara Walker, in *The Crone,* mentions the "old fashioned sewing circles and quilting bees" as bonding places for women.[13] The quilt itself, soft, made from homemade materials, lies in sharp contrast to the Vietnam monument and other memorials erected in Washington. AIDS masses—gathering around the Table, holy drink from a chalice—have evoked the feminine.

A powerful symbol of Mary emerged as I watched "A Gift of Grace," the story of Michael Prouty's spiritual journey with AIDS through his paintings, a videotape shown at General Convention. One of his paintings, *Soul Portrait,* has the gestalt of Madonna and Child and the suffering Christ at the same time. Prouty, near death, saw this himself, too. The figure wears a mask to show "the suffering I feel, rather than what I see," Prouty says. The

hands bear the stigmata and the figure is cradling an artist's palette like a child: "And the palette that he's holding is like a child
because I feel like my paintings are my legacy rather than the
having of children, so that's why the palette is being cradled like
a child."[14]

Though we have all experienced the "rejecting mothers" of
PWAs, so many others have nurtured. As I have read accounts of
caregiving mothers to sons, and as I have witnessed these in the
hospital, the image, the cairn of Michelangelo's *Pietà* intruded.
Barbara Peabody's *Screaming Room* is one such account.[15] Another is the final story included in this chapter. It is hard not to
see "God as Mother" while watching a caregiver, male or female,
tending a suffering person with the love of the best kind of
mother.

However, as I read further into feminist theology, I begin to
understand the question Monica Furlong poses in *Thérèse of
Lisieux:*

> Quite why women should be drawn to a religion that
> treated them so woundingly is an interesting question.
> Perhaps on the deepest level they understood Christianity
> better than it officially understood itself, and were nour-
> ished and comforted by it as the black slaves in America
> would come to be comforted by it in a society that had no
> human place for them at all. Forbidden all leadership, not
> permitted to raise their voices in public, to perform rites,
> to preach or teach, women still clung to the religion
> which spoke of love, sharing, and compassion, faithful in
> prayer, religious devotions, and acts of charity.[16]

I thought of how far women have come historically, but I also
remembered my own experience at General Convention. Ap-
pointed to the Social and Urban Committee in the House of
Deputies at General Convention, I was asked to chair the subcommittee on AIDS resolutions, perhaps from my own clinical
work as well as my position on the diocesan AIDS task force.
NEAC contacted me prior to Convention with their package;
other resolutions related to AIDS were also sent. Though I felt
inadequate to the task, I did my homework. I contacted the
NEAC booth prior to Convention and felt a solidarity with workers there similar to what I felt in Mississippi in the 1960s with
those working in civil rights.

I was not prepared, however, for the first day of our committee meeting when members were asked to select a subcommittee. No one joined mine. An AIDS subcommittee of one! Later two others did offer help, both women, and NEAC members followed the progress of resolutions, answered questions, or made suggestions as appropriate. When the day came for open hearings on AIDS in our committee (at 7 A.M., hardly a time to swell a crowd!), the NEAC provided a full contingent of speakers. Authors of other resolutions spoke, too. The reaction later from the whole committee was overwhelming. In the process, some were converted from fear or indifference to support.

The AIDS Healing Service occurred the next day; the AIDS Quilt had arrived and turned the basement of Cobo Hall into veritable catacombs beneath the House of Deputies. The AIDS resolutions came out of committee strategically, some alone, some in package. My greatest fear was that I would have to speak on the floor of that large assembly, to argue for explicit prevention education or compassionate caring. Within my notebook (my "scrapbag") were articles, statistics, and a story from the mother of a PWA.

I did speak on the floor of the house to give the rationale for one resolution. In addition, I asked the house to support our own bishops as they answered the presiding bishop's call for personal involvement in the life of a PWA for the following year. I suggested further that we, as deputies, do the same.

I was totally unprepared for two things that followed. The first was the passage of all AIDS resolutions, easily, effortlessly. The second was somewhat different. I heard later of a deputy from another southern diocese who said, after I had spoken, "That's the trouble with ordaining women; they always side with the underdog. Those people make me sick." I heard the remark as a gift but realized it also marked the great distance toward acceptance women must travel.

On return from General Convention, I reflected on the involvement of women in AIDS ministries, talked with several in neighboring cities, and have concluded that homophobia and "thanatophobia" do lie beneath the fears of many males, lay and ordained, who choose not to work with PWAs. Although I initially recoiled from Ogle's statement that "the root of homophobia is sexism," I find that I agree, albeit painfully. All I could think of was the AIDS Quilt panel with the words (also recalled in Bishop William Swing's sermon at the AIDS Healing Service), "Heal AIDS with love," part of the message from the last story in this paper.

The following piece, from "the absent panel member" who felt she could not attend our diocesan AIDS conference in Mississippi, is a separate panel in my proposed quilt. The conference for which this was written was cancelled for lack of interest; and although I had the writer's permission to read it at General Convention, should the occasion arise, I never did. Thus it lies, with several other stories, in my own scrap bag, finally open.

From the Absent Panel Member

I was asked to participate in this panel because I am the mother of a son who died of AIDS. I am also a physician and perhaps those who asked thought I might have some objectivity in this situation and could perhaps help the task force. I have no objectivity; I am just a woman who has lost her beloved son. Ask any woman who has experienced this and the loss is the same no matter what the cause. You expect your parents to die before you do but losing a child is "out of synch" as someone told me, and it is very bad. All I could offer would be a sad woman crying intermittently, so I turn down the offer to appear before you.

I am comforted by thinking of his life, not his death. His life in which he triumphed over his inner personal devils which he covered with alcohol and drugs for years, led him and me to a real faith. He found new life through honesty and a belief in God as he understood him. He carried in his wallet for seven years a piece of paper on which he had written: "If God loves me, who am I not to love myself?"

So I do have a message for this task force:

1. Tell the truth; teach people the facts about this horrible disastrous disease. Stop it; prevent it.

2. Never forget the real mission of the church, at least as I see it, acceptance of all God's people wherever they are, whatever their condition in this life. It has been through the love, caring, and support of friends, priests and God's grace that we carry on.

With her permission I wrote her son's name on the canvas

quilt at the NEAC booth and saw his life blessed in the Healing Service at General Convention. Like Ogle, I was totally unprepared for the feelings I had at that service and for the rare privilege of participating in the laying on of hands. The image of Michelangelo's *Pietà* intrudes here from the memory of her holding her son in the intensive care unit as the family prayed together at the time of death and from her words about "my beloved son."

Were I to make this piece into a panel for the quilt it would have an outline of the *Pietà* and, piercing into the limp body, red lines from IV poles, from Christ on the cross, and from a chalice. Bright sun would be overall.

Conclusion

An editorial in *The Internist* recently asked the question, "Can There Be a Bright Side to AIDS?" and answered affirmatively in several areas related to streamlining the regulatory systems for experimental drug tests and the possibilities for discoveries in research.[17] The editor noted that the atomic research during World War II that led to the violence of Hiroshima and Nagasaki also led to what we know now as nuclear medicine; there is hope for advances in all areas related to immunology as AIDS research proceeds.

But is the stone really rolled away? Is there hope in all of this? Yes, I think so. There is hope in a church that calls for compassion and presence. There is hope in a church where the presiding bishop announces that he, too, will become a "buddy" of a PWA. There is hope in a church that stops in its business week at General Convention for a healing service for PWAs. There is hope in a church that asks for dialogue, not debate, among *all* people within its structures. There is hope for a church that searches the issues, as we are doing in these essays.

But even more there is the hope that all of our lives offer, all of us called to work the fields in this pandemic. As we share our stories—even the broken ones—we begin to find the truth of the Incarnation, of grace affirmed, and of the power of the Holy Spirit that sustains and helps us stand in the dawning light of the resurrection with the great "cairn" rolled away. We have learned from the many lives and deaths of persons with AIDS more than we ever knew.

Like graves, we heal over, and yet keep
as part of ourselves the severe gift.
By grief, more inward than darkness,

the dead become the intelligence of life.
Where the tree falls and the forest rises.
there is nowhere to stand but in absence,
no life but in the fateful light.[18]

References

1. W. Berry, "Rising," in *Three Memorial Poems* (Berkeley, Calif.: Sand Dollar Books, 1977), p. 25.
2. J. Booty, *The Episcopal Church in Crisis* (Cambridge, Mass.: Cowley Publications, 1988), p. 9.
3. L. Kramer, *The Normal Heart* (New York: New American Books, 1985), p. 117.
4. F. Kivengere (Homily delivered at the Triennial Meeting of the Episcopal Church Women, September 14, 1979, in Denver, Colorado); from the personal notes of Ruth W. Black.
5. D. Tutu, *Hope and Suffering: Sermons and Speeches* (Grand Rapids, Mich.: Eerdmans, 1983), p. 187.
6. M. Muggeridge, *Something Beautiful for God: Mother Theresa of Calcutta* (Garden City, N.Y.: Image Books, 1977).
7. J. Fortunato, *AIDS: The Spiritual Dilemma* (San Francisco: Harper & Row, 1987), p. 100.
8. Fowler's theory is best applied in his *Faith Development and Pastoral Care* (Philadelphia: Fortress Press, 1987).
9. R. Reuther, *Womanguides: Readings toward a Feminist Theology* (Boston: Beacon Press, 1985).
10. C. Ruskin, *The Quilt: Stories from the NAMES Project* (New York: Pocket Books, 1988).
11. L. Nungesser, *Epidemic of Courage: Facing AIDS in America* (New York: St. Martin's Press, 1986).
12. N.A. Peete, "Reflections of an Episcopal Priest: In the Fullness of Time," *The Witness* (September 1988): pp. 16, 17.
13. B. Walker, *The Crone: Woman of Age, Wisdom, and Power* (San Francisco: Harper & Row, 1985).
14. For information regarding Michael Prouty and his work, contact Art For Innerpeace, 249 N. Brand Boulevard, Suite 584, Glendale, CA 91203. Telephone (213) 669–0140.

15. B. Peabody, *Screaming Room: A Mother's Journal of Her Son's Struggle with AIDS—A True Story of Love, Dedication, and Courage* (New York: Avon Books, 1986).
16. M. Furlong, *Thérèse of Lisieux* (New York: Pantheon Books, 1987), p. 4.
17. C. Burns Roehrig, M.D. "Can There Be a Bright Side to AIDS?" *The Internist,* Volume XXIX, No. 7, August 1988, p. 7.
18. Berry, *Three Memorial Poems,* p. 26.

Biographical Note

Ruth Black is a priest of the Diocese of Mississippi, serving as chaplain at the University of Mississippi Medical Center, where she is also a clinical instructor in the department of psychiatry. She earned her baccalaureate degree at Belhaven College in Jackson and her doctorate at Harvard University in language and literature. She was ordained deacon in 1986 and priest in 1987 in St. Andrew's Cathedral in Jackson. She is on the adjunct faculty at Millsaps College and, prior to entering holy orders, had a career as an educator at Millsaps College and Mississippi State University. She holds many positions in the Diocese of Mississippi, including membership on the diocesan AIDS commission.

Toward a Public Theology

J. Robert Brown

Albert Ogle deals with a number of issues related to the theology undergirding our response to AIDS. What strikes me most about his approach is that it provokes us to new ways of thinking about God and society.

The Church's ministry of healing too often has stressed the dispensation of healing power by healthy, active ministers to sick, passive objects of our concern. Ogle encourages us to turn that around—and meanwhile to turn ourselves—so that we may see the face of God in the face of a public health crisis. This means less emphasis on ministry to people with AIDS and a new appreciation of their ministry among us. This reorientation also means seeing the PWA as an active agent of healing ministry in the world.

AIDS makes us take a hard look at ourselves to examine our own attitudes toward sickness, sexuality, and death. It makes us take a critical look at a society that rejects people with AIDS while perpetuating a health care system on the brink of collapse. Ogle challenges us to rediscover story, cult, and symbol, the rich resources of our tradition that can be brought to bear on the AIDS crisis.

AIDS disproportionately affects minorities, the poor, and the oppressed, those Jesus calls God's "little ones": gay men, drug abusers, prostitutes, children newly born to AIDS-infected women. These are despised and rejected groups who, we are told, deserve to pay the consequences of their "life-style." Precisely for this reason the Church *must* stand in solidarity with these groups. It is essential for Christians to speak on behalf of victims of injustice and to protect vulnerable minorities from the bigotry of the majority. Now that AIDS is hitting the black and Hispanic communities particularly hard, it is becoming more apparent that AIDS is a "minority" issue.

Ogle is farsighted to include reference to the overcoming of "patriarchy"; in freeing the oppressor, all may be free. AIDS is a highly charged political issue that prominently raises questions about heterosexism and racism and, more subtly, about the sexism that lies at the root of both. As long as our images of God reinforce oppressive patterns of behavior, the Church will fall short of the unity God intends for his children.

"Transformation: Visions and Plans" calls us to that liberty and newness of life that is in store for us. We are like Lazarus raised from the grave, stumbling and nearly blinded by the light of new life. Let us hear our Lord's command: "Unbind him, and let him go free."

I read Ogle not only from the perspective of a priest but also from my position as a congressional legislative assistant. Those of us who have been involved in the development of legislation dealing with this issue are aware that, in spite of the inadequacies of the governmental response, some of the values we hold dear are at last "becoming flesh" in the public policy at the federal, state, and local level.

Probably the most intriguing part of working in the House of Representatives is seeing the clash of competing interests and values that somehow work together in the formation of public policy. My boss is a member of the Energy and Commerce Committee, which has jurisdiction over health legislation; he was a sponsor of the AIDS Federal Policy Act before signing on as a supporter became fashionable. As this is written (October 1988) that bill (now H.R. 5142) has passed both chambers and, if signed by the president, will become public law. The main provisions are remarkably enlightened in approaching testing and counseling, confidentiality of testing data, notification to emergency response employees, and support of AIDS research. However, it became clear that the "antidiscriminatory" provisions would have to be removed if the other parts were going to make it through the 100th Congress.

While we are hoping that federal antidiscriminatory legislation will be adopted in the next Congress, the protections against discrimination were still too controversial to become law this time around. This resistance—or at least reluctance—to adopt the antidiscriminatory legislation is revealing. It expresses the irrational fear that still affects public policy and keeps us from adopting a sound federal AIDS policy.

In spite of the setbacks, I have been impressed by the way we as a nation have grown in response to AIDS. The legislative correspondence about AIDS from "back home" in our congressional district has changed dramatically over the last two years. The letters have moved from frightened, bigoted, and bizarre to rational, sensible, and even compassionate.

When an antibody-positive child was admitted to a rural school in our district, we were expecting the worst; but the school board directed that the child be admitted; the principal and teachers set a sane tone, and the community rallied to the child's support. In rural Oklahoma, neighbors are still considered "kith and kin," and those folks weren't going to stand for anything that would hurt that student or his family.

While we see real advances in the strangest places, there have been discouraging setbacks "within the beltway" in our nation's capital. The city ordinance protecting people from discrimination in insurance on the basis of antibody status has been repealed, at the direction of Congress. A rider to the appropriations bill for the District of Columbia also directed the city council to amend the Human Rights Act to allow churches to discriminate against gays and lesbians. The move forward in public policy is in baby steps, generally moving in the right direction but too often also stumbling backward.

I have recently become a volunteer in the National Institutes of Health research for a vaccine. While being part of that effort is exciting, I realize that if the vaccine works as planned I will convert to antibody positive very shortly, joining the ranks of those stigmatized by their antibody status, in insurance, possibly in employment, and in other areas. While I expect to enjoy excellent health for many years to come, I'm going to be "kith and kin" in a new way.

So I end my remarks on public policy from that personal perspective, in the hope that the Word—the values of justice, compassion, and common sense—may become flesh in the public policy adopted at a federal, state, and local level. You and I will be instrumental in shaping that policy because we will shape public attitudes. That is a responsibility that is "moral," "theological," and "political" at one and the same time.

Biographical Note

John Robert Brown is legislative aid to the Honorable Mike Synar, Democrat of Oklahoma, in the House of Representatives. He earned his baccalaureate degree at the University of the South, a master's degree from Cambridge, and a theological degree from the General Theological Seminary. He also earned a master's in theology from Union Theological Seminary in New York and is a licentiate in sacred theology from the University of Louvain. He earned a diploma in ecumenical studies from the University of Geneva; he has done additional study at Harvard and Yale, and was a Fellow at the College of Preachers. He has had parochial experience in Oklahoma and Los Angeles.

Annotated Bibliography

Not surprisingly, recent years have seen a plethora of books published on the subject of acquired immune deficiency syndrome (AIDS). They range in quality from the superb to the execrable. This brief bibliography provides little more than a sampling, a general guideline. As with *Time* magazine's "Man of the Year," selection does not indicate approval. It is important to read the annotation accompanying each entry.

AIDS: Philosophical, Sociological

Aaron, Anne, and Iben Browning. *The Economic Impact of AIDS.* Sapiens Press, 1988. This book is a curious mixture of truth, half-truth, and no truth at all. The mixture makes the book a negative contribution to solving the problems of the AIDS crisis.

Bateson, Mary Catherine, and Richard Goldsby. *Thinking AIDS: The Social Response to the Biological Threat.* Reading, Mass.: Addison-Wesley Publishing, 1988. A wise and stimulating book that no one concerned with thinking about AIDS should miss. The authors present AIDS integratively as a biological, medical personal, social, and ethical reality in a fashion both learned and clear.

Dreuilhe, Emmanuel. Translated by Linda Coverdale. *Mortal Embrace: Living With AIDS.* New York: Hill and Wang, 1989. Using the metaphor of war, a multinational Frenchman contends that a foreign enemy, the AIDS virus, has declared war on the human race. This provocative reflection by a person with AIDS is critical of many religious leaders. Dreuilhe writes, "Even more than our immunity, it's our confidence that the virus has destroyed. We no longer believe in ourselves or in all those who have betrayed and deceived us. . . . For me, AIDS was first of all the experience of solitude." Does faith in God have something to say to this?

Hay, Louise L. *You Can Heal Your Life.* Santa Monica: Hay House, 1984; *The AIDS Book: Creating a Positive Approach,* Santa Monica: Hay House, 1988. Louise Hay has developed a large following; many attribute great things to her. While we can celebrate the healing effects of the caring community she has developed, her ideas regarding spiritual healing are appallingly simplistic. Though some people sing her praises, others are unable to bring about the cure that Hay promised would be available if they only adopted the correct attitudes: they often feel far worse than they did before encountering Hay. Her New Age philosophy has been described as a "kind of lite metaphysics that implies that, if you think right thoughts, and do right things, life is controllable. If, on the other hand, the Mysteriousness of God comes into play and you get an infection, it was probably your own fault." Avoid these books. She makes no claim to be a practitioner of Christian spiritual healing. Good. Her ideas are clearly un-Christian.

Kubler-Ross, Elisabeth. *AIDS: The Ultimate Challenge.* New York: Macmillan, 1987. One of the most disappointing of recent AIDS books, it seems pasted together and poorly structured.

Masters, William, Virginia Johnson, and Robert Kolodney. *Crisis: Heterosexual Behavior in the Age of AIDS.* New York: St. Martin's Press, 1988. This book is dangerous; its authors are well known, and they have earned credibility through their pioneering research into the physiology of human sexuality. However, this book contains misstatements of fact; its tone is alarmist. They have forfeited their right to their hard-earned credibility. Avoid this book.

Monette, Paul. *Borrowed Time: An AIDS Memoir.* San Diego: Harcourt/Brace/Jovanovich, 1988. This story of two men, one who dies, the other whose immune system is compromised, is a poignant study of denial, which is perhaps the most significant psychological feature of the AIDS crisis. This is an important narrative of the AIDS crisis.

Pierce, Christine, and Donald VanDeVeer, eds. *AIDS: Ethics and Public Policy.* Belmont, Calif.: Wadsworth, 1988. A solid collection of essays to support ethical discussion.

Shilts, Randy. *And the Band Played On: Politics, People, and the AIDS Epidemic.* New York: St. Martin's Press, 1987. This exhaustive chronological account of the AIDS epidemic is mandatory reading for any who wish to understand AIDS in relationship to American social and political culture and public policy.

Siegel, M.D., Bernie. *Love, Medicine, and Miracles.* New York: Harper & Row, 1986. This is a book about surviving, about survivors' characteristics, about healing medical insights, and about taking control in order to heal oneself. Siegel's views are integrative. He sees the human being as unitary and recognizes that spiritual health is of equal importance with (and inseparable from) physical health. Highly recommended.

Sontag, Susan. *Aids and Its Metaphors.* New York: Farrar, Straus & Giroux, 1989. Sontag urges us to use a different metaphor for AIDS, explaining that the dread metaphors of cancer degrade the experience of the patient, blame the victim, and contribute to demoralization. She also rejects the metaphors of war and invasion. The writing is sparkling, quirky, and tendentious. She provides an intellectualist account of the "idea" of AIDS.

AIDS: Theological, Spiritual

Countryman, Louis William. "The AIDS Crisis: Theological and Ethical Reflections." *Anglican Theological Review* 69(1987):125–34. An early effort to speak theologically to the issues. It may still be useful, especially as refuting notions of AIDS as punishment.

Fortunato, John. *AIDS: The Spiritual Dilemma.* San Francisco: Harper & Row, 1987. The author, an able lay theologian who is also a psychotherapist and a gay man, emphasizes the importance of embodiment and of the Christian hope of resurrection as we struggle with God's reality in the face of AIDS. Highly recommended.

Fortunato, John. *Embracing the Exile: Healing Journeys of Gay Christians.* Minneapolis: Winston/Seabury, 1982. Strictly speaking, this is not a book about AIDS but about spirituality, homosexuality, and psycho-spiritual wholeness. It is of immense value to Christians attempting to respond to gay people with AIDS.

Jones, William Closson, ed. *AIDS in Religious Perspective.* Papers by Paul R. Johnson, William P. Zion, and Bruce L. Mills. Kingston, Ontario: Queen's Theological College, 1987. Three academic papers here offer useful and provocative insights into the ethical analysis of AIDS issues, the theological background of the churches' responses, and the psychology of homophobia and AIDS panic.

Religious Education (Spring 1988). This issue contains a collection of articles entitled "AIDS: Sexual Responsibility and

Ethics." These vary widely in terms of presuppositions and quality. Those by Charles R. McCarthy (a physician's plea for action on the part of America's churches) and by Karen Lebacqz and Deborah Blake ("Safe Sex and Lost Love") are particularly good. This collection is useful for exploring sexual ethics, AIDS education, and related issues.

Smith, S.J., Walter J. *AIDS: Living and Dying with Hope: Issues in Pastoral Care.* Ramsey, N.J. Paulist Press, 1988. A thoughtful book by a compassionate Roman Catholic.

Snow, John. *Mortal Fear: Meditations on Death and AIDS.* Cambridge, Mass.: Cowley Publications, 1987. A professor at the Episcopal Divinity School writes five short meditations on the significance of AIDS and three somewhat longer ones on the meaning of death in our time. The style is clear and the contents serious and helpful.

AIDS and the Church's Response

Amos, Jr., William E. *When AIDS Comes to Church.* Philadelphia: Westminster Press, 1988. A solid, if somewhat conservative, introduction to AIDS ministry by a Baptist pastor from Florida.

Christianity and Crisis 48(July 4, 1988). This special issue on AIDS is an excellent collection of current articles and a great resource for an adult education class.

Kirkpatrick, Bill. *AIDS: Sharing the Pain: Pastoral Guidelines.* London: Darton, Longman and Todd. 1988. A wise book by an Anglican priest who has spearheaded AIDS work in London.

Shelp, Earl E., and Ronald H. Sunderland. *AIDS and the Church.* Philadelphia: Westminster Press, 1987. A superb introduction to AIDS ministry issues.

AIDS: Practical Care

Alyson, Sasha, ed. *You CAN Do Something About AIDS.* Boston: Stop AIDS Project (40 Plympton St., Boston, MA 02118), 1988. This little volume is a project of the publishing industry and was distributed without charge by the Book of the Month Club. It is a compilation of essays about activist projects during the AIDS crisis and includes a useful list of resources.

Hughes, A., J. Martin, and P. Franks. *AIDS Home Care and Hospice Manual.* San Francisco: Visiting Nurse Association of

San Francisco, 1987. A useful "how to" book.

Martelli, Leonard J., with Fran D. Peltz, C.R.C., and William Messina, C.S.W. *When Someone You Know Has AIDS: A Practical Guide.* New York: Crown Publishers, 1987. With warm and compassionate narratives and first-person accounts, the authors provide a factual précis on dealing with the tragedy of AIDS. It is not so much a work on how to die as it is one on how to be human. Highly recommended.

Moffatt, M.A., Betty Clare, Judith Spiegle, M.P.H., Steve Parrish, and Michael Helquist, Eds. *AIDS: A Self Care Manual.* Santa Monica, Calif.: IBS Press, 1987. A comprehensive book, this includes a solid section on the spiritual and religious dimensions of AIDS.

Human Sexuality: General

Bell, Alan P., and Martin S. Weinberg. *Homosexualities: A Study of Diversity among Men and Women.* New York: Simon & Schuster, 1978. This is the first book based upon the extensive interview research conducted in the homophile community by the Kinsey Institute for Sex Research and is essential reading for those interested in the phenomenon of homosexuality. The following book is further analysis of the same research.

Bell, Alan P., Martin S. Weinberg, and Susan K. Hammersmith. *Sexual Preference: Its Development in Men and Women.* Bloomington: Indiana University Press, 1981. This is the most authoritative study of the phenomenon of sex object orientation available, based on analysis of extensive research conducted over many years by the Kinsey Institute for Sex Research.

Human Sexuality: Theological

Batchelor, Jr., Edward, ed. *Homosexuality and Ethics.* New York: Pilgrim Press, 1980. This is a symposium with contributions, most previously published, from such distinguished contributors as Roger Shinn, Tom Driver, Gregory Baum, Rosemary Ruether, Aquinas, Barth, Curran, Thielicke, and Lisa Sowle Cahill. It has the advantage of a variety of perspectives and is also, predictably, uneven. Sadly, an essay by priest-psychiatrist Ruth Tiffany Barnhouse has been included, although her perspective on homosexuality is seen as gravely flawed by both her Jungian colleagues and most students of human sexuality. An excellent source book.

Boswell, John. *Christianity, Social Tolerance, and Homosexuality: Gay People in Western Europe from the Beginning of the Christian Era to the Fourteenth Century.* Chicago: University of Chicago Press, 1980. Winner of the 1981 American Book Award for history, this volume is a rarity, combining scholarly erudition with a quality of fascination that prevents many readers from putting it down until finished. Boswell is a virtuoso student of history, languages, the Bible, and ancient literature. His observations about the prejudices of translators and illustrations of how their biases have shaped our thinking are of immense importance to us during the AIDS crisis.

Cole, William Graham. *Sex in Christianity and Psychoanalysis.* New York: Oxford University Press, 1966. Regrettably, this book is out of print but may be available in a library. The author, a pioneer in efforts to have sex education in the churches, is a Presbyterian clergyman and college professor and president. He has written a valuable book that connects interpretations of sex in Christianity and psychoanalysis, concluding with "a critical reconstruction of Christian interpretations of sex." Very helpful.

Cole, William Graham. *Sex and Love in the Bible.* London: Hodder and Stoughton, 1960. This is a forthright presentation of all major Old and New Testament incidents, attitudes, and precepts involving sex and love, from the Genesis accounts of Adam and Eve to St. Paul's comments on marital love obligations.

Countryman, Louis William. *Dirt, Greed, and Sex: Sexual Ethics in the New Testament and Their Implications for Today.* Philadelphia: Fortress Press, 1988. Presents a new exegesis and interpretation of New Testament passages pertaining to homosexual acts.

Horner, Tom. *Jonathan Loved David: Homosexuality in Biblical Times.* Philadelphia: Westminster Press, 1978. Horner provides a scholarly accounting of cultural/sexual values in the Middle East during the two millennia prior to the common era, then presents an exposition on the relationship of David and Jonathan, and Ruth and Naomi, as well as the stories of Sodom and Gibeah. The last three chapters deal with the writings of Paul and "Jesus and Sexuality." The book is well equipped with scholarly apparatus. Recommended for specialists and scholars.

Kosnick, Anthony, and the Catholic Theological Society of America. *Human Sexuality: New Directions in American*

Catholic Thought. New York: Paulist Press, 1977. The CTSA is an organization deserving high respect. It functions independently of the Roman Catholic hierarchy. It commissioned the studies included in this volume and was hailed by critics as a landmark contribution to the study of sexuality, theology, and pastoral care. It is a great tragedy that the book was denounced by the hierarchy, which imposed *a priori* assumptions on the studies, which were, in the tradition of good scholarship, ignored by its authors. Highly recommended.

McNeill, S.J., John J. *The Church and the Homosexual.* Kansas City: Sheed Andrews and McMeel, 1976. McNeill has paid a high price for his courageous scholarship and advocacy since he first published this excellent book. His relationship with the Roman Catholic Church and the Society of Jesus has been turbulent in the intervening years. His book deals with moral theology, Scripture, tradition, pastoral care, and justice and the homosexual. An important book.

Nelson, James B. *Embodiment: An Approach to Sexuality and Christian Theology.* Minneapolis: Augsburg, 1978. Nelson, a professor of theology at United Theological Seminary of the Twin Cities, has written a book useful in seminaries and local congregations as a safe introduction to this subject, seen as frightening by so many. The book has proved its value during its first decade.

Sapp, Stephen. *Sexuality, the Bible, and Science.* Philadelphia: Fortress Press, 1977. A noted United Methodist teacher and clergyman approaches sexuality from a biblical perspective, harmonizing the ancient narratives with a contemporary scientific approach to produce a dialectical view of human sexuality. A very valuable book.

Scroggs, Robin. *The New Testament and Homosexuality: Contextual Background for Contemporary Debate.* Philadelphia: Fortress Press, 1983. This moderate and cautious book examines closely the use of the Scriptures in the contemporary Church and provides a context for understanding references to homosexual activity in the New Testament. Scroggs, a seminary professor, reviews Palestinian Judaism, Hellenistic Judaism, the early Church, and their views of homosexuality. His thoughtful approach, supported by good appendices and indices, makes this a valuable contribution to this topic.

Spong, John Shelby. *Living in Sin: A Bishop Rethinks Hu-*

man Sexuality. San Francisco: Harper & Row, 1988. This controversial book by a controversial bishop reiterates the issues of biblical study, theology of sexuality, sociology of homosexuality, and ethics that have been thoroughly explored by other scholars, some listed in this bibliography. Spong has devised a synthesis that is "shocking" only because it is articulated by bishop. From a scholarly point of view this book is in the mainstream of progressive thought. It is flawed, not only by its unfortunate title, but more importantly by the lack of footnotes and other scholarly apparatus. Many people sympathetic with the book may take issue with Spong's proposals about the church blessing of gay unions, but it is valuable nonetheless. Very useful as a discussion vehicle.

Death

Humphry, Derek. *Let Me Die Before I Wake. Hemlock's Book of Self-Deliverance for the Dying.* New York: Hemlock Society/ Grove Press, 1985. Those who work with persons with AIDS need to know what is in this book, even if they disagree with every idea. The Hemlock Society supports the right of terminally ill people to practice "self-deliverance," and this book includes many moving stories of people who have chosen to do that. It includes an essay titled "Some social aspects of terminal illness," by ethicist Gerald A. Larue, as well as examples of a durable power of attorney and a "living will." It is a useful resource book, and is very germane to those living with AIDS.

Becker, Ernest. *The Denial of Death.* New York: Free Press (Macmillan), 1973. Cited in this book by Ted Karpf, this is a serious and valuable scholarly study.

Kubler-Ross, Elisabeth. *On Death and Dying.* New York: Macmillan, 1976. By now this is probably the best known book on the subject. It is accessible, and has been of great value to many.

Schneidman, Edwin S. *Death: Current Perspectives.* Palo Alto, Calif., Mayfield, 1984. Schneidman may be America's preeminent authority on death. A professor at University of California, Los Angeles, his classes are very popular, and his books invariably cited in connection with the psychology of death.